DRUGS
The Straight Facts

Prescription
Pain Relievers

DRUGS The Straight Facts

■ DRUGS
The Straight Facts

Prescription Pain Relievers

M. Foster Olive

Consulting Editor

David J. Triggle

University Professor
School of Pharmacy and Pharmaceutical Sciences
State University of New York at Buffalo

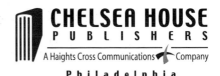

CHELSEA HOUSE
P U B L I S H E R S
A Haights Cross Communications Company
Philadelphia

CHELSEA HOUSE PUBLISHERS
VP, New Product Development Sally Cheney
Director of Production Kim Shinners
Creative Manager Takeshi Takahashi
Manufacturing Manager Diann Grasse

Staff for PRESCRIPTION PAIN RELIEVERS
Executive Editor Tara Koellhoffer
Associate Editor Beth Reger
Editorial Assistant Kuorkor Dzani
Production Editor Noelle Nardone
Photo Editor Sarah Bloom
Series & Cover Designer Terry Mallon
Layout 21st Century Publishing and Communications, Inc.

A Haights Cross Communications ◄— Company

http://www.chelseahouse.com

First Printing

1 3 5 7 9 8 6 4 2

Library of Congress Cataloging-in-Publication Data

Olive, M. Foster.
  Prescription Pain relievers/M. Foster Olive.
    p. cm.—(Drugs, the straight facts)
  ISBN 0-7910-8199-0 — ISBN 0-7910-8375-6 (pbk.)
  1. Analgesics—Juvenile literature. I. Title. II. Series.
RM319.O455 2004
615'.783—dc22

                                        2004024372

All links and web addresses were checked and verified to be correct at the time
of publication. Because of the dynamic nature of the web, some addresses and
links may have changed since publication and may no longer be valid.

Table of Contents

The Use and Abuse of Drugs

The issues associated with drug use and abuse in contemporary society are vexing subjects, fraught with political agendas and ideals that often obscure essential information that teens need to know to have intelligent discussions about how to best deal with the problems associated with drug use and abuse. *Drugs: The Straight Facts* aims to provide this essential information through straightforward explanations of how an individual drug or group of drugs works in both therapeutic and non-therapeutic conditions; with historical information about the use and abuse of specific drugs; with discussion of drug policies in the United States; and with an ample list of further reading.

From the start, the series uses the word *"drug"* to describe psychoactive substances that are used for medicinal or non-medicinal purposes. Included in this broad category are substances that are legal or illegal. It is worth noting that humans have used many of these substances for hundreds, if not thousands of years. For example, traces of marijuana and cocaine have been found in Egyptian mummies; the use of peyote and Amanita fungi has long been a component of religious ceremonies worldwide; and alcohol production and consumption have been an integral part of many human cultures' social and religious ceremonies. One can speculate about why early human societies chose to use such drugs. Perhaps, anything that could provide relief from the harshness of life—anything that could make the poor conditions and fatigue associated with hard work easier to bear—was considered a welcome tonic. Life was likely to be, according to the seventeenth century English philosopher Thomas Hobbes, *"poor, nasty, brutish and short."* One can also speculate about modern human societies' continued use and abuse of drugs. Whatever the reasons, the consequences of sustained drug use are not insignificant—addiction, overdose, incarceration, and drug wars—and must be dealt with by an informed citizenry.

The problem that faces our society today is how to break

the connection between our demand for drugs and the willingness of largely outside countries to supply this highly profitable trade. This is the same problem we have faced since narcotics and cocaine were outlawed by the Harrison Narcotic Act of 1914, and we have yet to defeat it despite current expenditures of approximately $20 billion per year on "the war on drugs." The first step in meeting any challenge is always an intelligent and informed citizenry. The purpose of this series is to educate our readers so that they can make informed decisions about issues related to drugs and drug abuse.

SUGGESTED ADDITIONAL READING

David T. Courtwright, *Forces of Habit. Drugs and the Making of the Modern World.* Cambridge, Mass.: Harvard University Press, 2001. David Courtwright is Professor of History at the University of North Florida.

Richard Davenport-Hines, *The Pursuit of Oblivion. A Global History of Narcotics.* New York: Norton, 2002. The author is a professional historian and a member of the Royal Historical Society.

Aldous Huxley, *Brave New World.* New York: Harper & Row, 1932. Huxley's book, written in 1932, paints a picture of a cloned society devoted only to the pursuit of happiness.

David J. Triggle, Ph.D.
University Professor
School of Pharmacy and Pharmaceutical Sciences
State University of New York at Buffalo

1

How Pain Works

Pain (noun): physical or mental suffering or distress, especially an unpleasant sensation arising from injury or disease.

—Merriam-Webster's Dictionary

We have all felt it, and we probably agree that of all the sensations we are capable of experiencing, pain is our least favorite. Sometimes it's a shooting pain, like when we step barefoot on a nail or accidentally bite our tongue. Sometimes it comes on very slowly and lingers for hours or days, like a bad sunburn. Or it might hurt only when we move a part of our body, like after we pull a hamstring or sprain an ankle. Still other times, such as during a migraine, the pain comes and goes, with days, weeks, or months between episodes; when it does come, it leaves us almost incapable of functioning.

Other than pain, few sensations have generated so many words in the English language to describe them. Pain can be dull, nagging, sharp, burning, aching, searing, gnawing, scalding, stinging, crushing, pulsing, throbbing, pounding, shooting, pricking, stabbing, cramping, wrenching, splitting, unbearable, excruciating, agonizing, blinding, grueling—pick your favorite.

WHY DO WE FEEL PAIN?
Since we all pretty much hate pain, why do we feel it? What "good" can come from it? The truth is that pain is very, *very* helpful to us. Humans as a species would likely not have survived very long without the sensation of pain. Pain tells us when something is injuring or damaging our skin, muscle, and other tissues and organs.

For example, pain keeps us from burning our hands when lighting a match or starting a fire. Pain tells us we might have a cavity in a tooth or a more serious problem in our teeth (mention the words *root canal* and most people shudder with fear). Stomach pain tells us we may have eaten something poisonous or that we may have an ulcer. Chest pain tells us we may be having a heart attack. Pain rapidly gets our attention, and we immediately look for ways to get rid of it. Because of pain, we are able to avoid hurting ourselves and damaging our tissues and organs, and we become aware of possible diseases that we may have.

PAIN SHAPES OUR BEHAVIOR

We may or may not accept that pain is a very helpful sensation, but most of us develop a natural *fear* of pain. We subsequently shape much of our own behavior around avoiding pain. We avoid places, situations, or objects that we associate with previously painful experiences. We avoid the dentist so we don't have to experience that horrible metal hook that probes and pokes around in our mouth for what seems like an eternity. Or, we avoid the allergist because of the needle that we think looks and feels like the size of a whale harpoon. Although these "doctor phobia" avoidance behaviors may not be in the best interest of our overall health, there are some pain-avoiding behaviors from which we can benefit. And we need not even have experienced the particular type of pain to avoid such situations. For example, some of us avoid heights because of a fear of falling off the edge of a cliff or building and the pain that would certainly follow, even though we have probably never actually fallen off a cliff or building. We do not walk in the middle of busy streets for fear of getting hit by a car and enduring severe pain or death, even though we may never have been hit by a car in real life. Common sense tells us to avoid pain. We avoid it sometimes by instinct, sometimes by learning from experience, and sometimes by learning from the misfortunes of others. Have you ever seen

(continued on page 12)

WHEN WE DON'T FEEL PAIN AT MOMENTS WE EXPECT IT THE MOST

Pain can act in strange ways. Many people suffer traumatic injuries but later state that, at the time, they felt no pain at all. For example, on March 30, 1981, John Hinckley, Jr., attempted to assassinate President Ronald Reagan with a handgun. When the gunshots were fired, President Reagan's aides pushed him into his limousine to protect him and then sped off. No one, not even President Reagan, knew immediately that he had been shot in the chest with a 9-mm bullet. A few moments later, President Reagan slumped against the car door and felt blood pouring from his chest. Only then did he start to feel excruciating pain. Up until that point, he had felt no pain at all.[1]

Another example took place on New Year's Eve, 1984. Rick Allen (Figure 1.1), a drummer for the hard rock band Def Leppard, was driving in his Corvette through the English countryside late at night and miscalculated a sharp turn, rolling his car over and smashing into a stone wall. Allen was thrown out of the car through the sunroof and landed in a field. After a brief blackout, he awoke, stood in the field, and realized that his left arm had been completely torn off—it had been held in place by the car's seatbelt. At the time, he felt no pain whatsoever.[2] Military personnel have told similar stories after losing a limb from an exploding mortar shell or land mine. No pain.

How is it that the mind senses severe pain immediately after getting a door slammed on the fingers, but can feel nothing after being shot in the chest or having an entire limb severed from the body? Scientists and doctors are not sure, because most reports about this are anecdotal and there is no way to examine such experiences in a controlled laboratory setting. But neuroscientists believe that the brain's ability to sense pain can turn off in times of shock and extreme

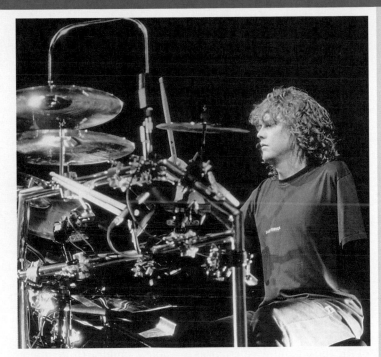

Figure 1.1 *Rick Allen, the drummer for the rock band Def Leppard, lost his arm in an automobile accident. He reports that, at the time of the accident, he did not feel any pain. Preventing the feeling of pain under extreme circumstances is just one of the mysteries of the brain and the body.*

emotional distress, offering the advantage of allowing the person to get out of a dangerous situation without being crippled by intense pain.

Sources:

1. Wall, P. *Pain: The Science of Suffering.* New York: Columbia University Press, 1999, p. 7.

2. Bradman, Mel. "Best of Times, Worst of Times: Rick Allen." *Sunday Times Magazine*, March 2, 2003. Available online at *http://www.angelfire.com/band/rickallenthundergod/sundaytimes.html.*

(continued from page 9)

someone smack his or her shin into a coffee table or bang a thumb with a hammer? We empathize with the painful experiences of others and learn to be more careful.

Pain is not purely a physiological process that is experienced the same way in every individual. The perception and tolerance of pain vary widely from person to person. Hollywood heroes such as James Bond, Rambo, and Rocky Balboa seem invincible to pain, but that's Hollywood. Everyone feels pain, but some have a greater tolerance to it than others. Cultural and psychological factors play a large role in how we experience pain, or at least how we show it. Many cultures, both ancient and modern, have ceremonies and rituals in which individuals (usually adolescent boys or young men) must endure extreme pain and physical demands without emitting so much as a whimper in order to become an "adult," "man," or "soldier." In sports and athletics, pain is seen as something that strengthens our character, talents, and abilities. Hence, the phrase "No pain, no gain." Ironically, although the ability to endure intense pain has traditionally been viewed as characteristic of being a "man," it is women who endure one of the most painful experiences possible—childbirth. Yet there is no societal "promotion" or advancement given to women for going through such an excruciating event.

PAIN THAT KEEPS ON GIVING

We all experience *acute* (short-lived) pain sometime in our lives—a scratch, a paper cut, a hangnail, a fall from a bike, a sock from a baseball, a sprained ankle. Acute pain lasts from a few seconds to a few hours to a few weeks. Some acute pain can be recurrent, coming on for relatively short periods of time and revisiting at frequent intervals. The best example of acute recurrent pain is in people who suffer from recurrent migraine headaches. There is some debate about how to classify these recurrent pain syndromes such as migraine—whether they are acute or chronic pain, or both.

Fortunately, acute pain goes away relatively quickly, either on its own or with medication or other medical treatment. However, millions of people suffer from some form of pain that is *chronic* (i.e., it lasts for years, sometimes for most of the person's life). Chronic pain causes not only terrible suffering to the individual, but also severe economic and social consequences, such as the inability to work or spend time with family. Chronic pain often results in depression, addiction to pain medications, and, in rare instances, suicide. Below are some medical conditions that are characterized by chronic pain:

- **Amputation:** Occasionally, amputation of a limb is medically necessary after a traumatic accident or injury, to stop the spread of cancer, or to treat severe disease in a limb's tissue or blood vessels. When a limb is surgically removed, major nerve fibers that supplied the limb are severed. Initially after amputation, the patient feels (usually quite convincingly) that the limb is still attached. This is known as "phantom limb" syndrome. At first, this phantom limb phenomenon is not painful, but it can be very confusing to the patient. Over time, the nerve fibers that once supplied the now missing limb attempt to grow back into the limb, but they have nowhere to go, so they ultimately grow into various tangles. This creates tender spots on the limb stump. These newly sprouted nerve fibers can spontaneously and mistakenly send pain signals to the brain in the form of violent stabs or constant burning or cramping.

- **Arthritis:** Arthritis is the general term for chronic pain in the joints: the fingers, wrists, elbows, shoulders, knees, ankles, and feet. There are two types of arthritis— *rheumatoid arthritis*, which results from an inflammation of the thin membranes that line the joints, and the more common *osteoarthritis*, which results from a progressive breakdown of the cushions of cartilage between the bones. Both types of arthritis can be extremely painful and result in severe joint pain, stiffness, limited motion, and fatigue. Arthritis is most often found in the elderly and is usually treated with anti-inflammatory medications (see Chapters 2 and 4).

- **Backaches:** Almost everyone—even young people—has at some point experienced pain in the back, especially the lower back. This can result from over-straining while lifting a heavy object, from injury during sports, from sleeping on an uncomfortable surface, or from other causes. However, some back pains can be defined as chronic and take weeks, months, or even years to recover from. Back pain is usually caused by a compressed nerve, slipped vertebral disk, fracture of a vertebra, muscle strain, infection, tumor, or arthritis. It can result in an inability to sit, stand, or lie down comfortably and often alters a person's posture. Back pain is often treated with various medications described in this book, but also by chiropractic alignment, yoga, massage, and acupuncture methods.

- **Cancer:** Cancer cells are almost exactly like normal cells in the body, but they multiply out of control and cause tumors to form. These tumors eventually grow large enough to put pressure on nerve endings, blood vessels, air passages in the lungs, and the sensitive covering of bones. This causes pain. Cancer can also damage nerve fibers, and this nerve damage (called neuropathy) causes pain. However, not all cancers are painful. For example, smaller brain tumors are not painful because the brain itself cannot feel pain, despite being made up of billions of nerve cells! Only when the tumor becomes large enough to exert pressure on the skull or blood vessels surrounding the brain do brain tumors become chronically painful.

- **Carpal tunnel syndrome:** Sometimes called repetitive stress or motion injury, carpal tunnel syndrome (CTS) results from overuse and overly repetitive motions of the arms, hands, and fingers. The people who are affected are often those whose occupations require them to use repetitive hand or wrist motions, such as assembly-line workers, grocery store clerks, and computer programmers. CTS is caused by a compression, or entrapment, of the nerves, tendons, and blood vessels that flow from the forearm to the hand through a small tunnel (the carpal tunnel, formed by the carpal ligament) in the wrist. The person with CTS first feels numbness or tingling in the fingers and eventually pain that can radiate into the upper arm. Common treatments for CTS are immobilizing the wrist with a splint, changing work habits and/or ergonomics (i.e., using wrist rests with computer keyboards), surgery to reopen the carpal tunnel, and medications such as ibuprofen, cortisone, and lidocaine (discussed in Chapters 2, 4, and 5).

- **Headaches:** Although many people get so-called "tension" headaches, some people experience headaches so severe that they are barely able to think or function. The most common type of severe headache is migraine. Migraines affect 10–15% of the U.S. population and occur most often in women (75% of the time). Migraines tend to run in families as well. The precise cause of migraines is unknown, but it is suspected that inflammation or sudden dilation of the blood vessels and nerves surrounding the brain could be to blame. Migraines have many triggers, such as bright lights, certain foods, changes in weather or climate, alcohol, hormonal changes, hunger, stress, and lack of sleep.

Most sufferers describe a migraine as a throbbing or pulsating pain that starts in a specific area of the head and later spreads over the rest of the head. Migraines tend to intensify over a 1- to 2-hour period (sometimes longer), then gradually subside. People with migraines often feel nauseated and overly sensitive to light, sound, and odors. After the migraine passes, the sufferer is left feeling weak and drained. Some migraine sufferers experience an "aura" about 10–30 minutes before the onset of the migraine. An aura is the experience of bright shimmering lights in the peripheral (side) vision, wavy or zigzag lines, hallucinations, or muscle weakness or numbness. It is unknown how this aura relates to the cause or symptoms of a migraine. Medications to treat migraine are described in Chapter 4.

- **Fibromyalgia:** Fibromyalgia (fī"-brō-mī-al'-jēə) is a medical condition that causes widespread aching or burning pain in many parts of the body, such as the neck, shoulders, chest, back, hips, hands, and feet. An estimated 6–8 million Americans suffer from fibromyalgia, and 80% are women, primarily between the ages of 20 and 40. Most sufferers sleep poorly because of the constant pain, and they are fatigued and sleepy during the day. The pain is often worse in the morning, better during the day, then worse again at night. The cause of fibromyalgia is unknown but may involve a malfunction of the immune system or spinal cord. Fibromyalgia is often treated with narcotic pain relievers (see Chapter 3) or other prescription medications, such as amitriptyline and muscle relaxants (see Chapter 4).

- **Multiple sclerosis:** Often called MS, multiple sclerosis is caused by a progressive, gradual degeneration of myelin, a fatty substance that coats nerve fibers to increase the speed at which they conduct their electrical signals. This degeneration of myelin is thought to result from a malfunction of the immune system, in which immune cells make a mistake and attack the body's own myelin-producing cells. The result is scarring and hardening of nerve fibers in the spinal cord, brain stem, and optic nerves. As a consequence, nerve fibers carry signals more slowly. This can cause muscle weakness and stiffness, fatigue, numbness, bladder dysfunction, excessive pain, and loss of vision. MS is often treated with muscle relaxants (see Chapter 4) and steroids or other immuno-suppressants (see Chapter 5) to reduce inflammation.

- **Shingles:** We are not referring here to the kind of shingles you put on roofs. Shingles is a painful condition caused by the same virus that causes chicken pox. People who were exposed to the chicken pox virus as children often have small amounts of dormant virus particles around their spinal cord. For some reason, mainly in adults over age 50, stress, cancer, or infection with HIV can cause these chicken pox viruses to become active, multiply, and migrate along the nerve fibers that extend from the spinal cord to the skin. Here, the virus produces a temporary band of redness and inflammation, which subsequently dies down and forms scar tissue. However, this process can destroy some of the nerve endings in the skin, and the same process of nerve regrowth and subsequent chronic pain that is experienced by an amputee (see page 13) can happen to a person who has had shingles. In shingles, the pain is limited to these small bands of scar tissue. Antiviral medications, various pain relievers, and neurosurgical procedures are the treatments of choice for shingles.

- **Trigeminal neuralgia:** Trigeminal neuralgia, or tic douloureux (doo-loo-roo') is a relatively rare medical condition characterized by terrible pain in the face, particularly a stabbing sensation on one side that feels like an electric shock. These intense, painful episodes begin and end rather quickly. They occur equally in men and women, most often between the ages of 50 and 70. One would think that trigeminal neuralgia is the manifestation of something wrong with the trigeminal nerve (the major nerve that senses pain in the face), but doctors have yet to find anything obviously wrong with this nerve system in affected patients. Trigeminal neuralgia is commonly treated with anticonvulsant medications (see Chapter 4) or some type of surgical procedure on the trigeminal nerve.

PAIN TERMINOLOGY

The medical term for the perception of pain is *nociception* (pronounced nō'-sih-sep-shun), or the perception of noxious (unpleasant or painful) events. Thus, the nerve endings in the skin, muscles, and internal organs that respond to painful stimuli are called *nociceptors.* (Technically speaking, nociceptors are actually small proteins located on these nerve endings; however, for the purposes of this book, we will refer to these proteins or the nerve endings themselves as being nociceptors.) The process of reducing or eliminating pain without producing a loss of consciousness is called *analgesia*; thus, pain relievers are often called *analgesics.* Analgesia is different from *anesthesia*, which is the elimination of pain by producing a loss of consciousness, as is done when someone has major surgery. However, the terms *analgesic* and *anesthetic* (drugs or agents that produce analgesia and anesthesia, respectively) are often used interchangeably. Finally, the term *hyperalgesia* describes a state in which nonpainful stimuli, such as touching one's arm or moving a joint, becomes very painful because of inflammation or tissue damage. Examples of this are sunburned skin and a sprained ankle.

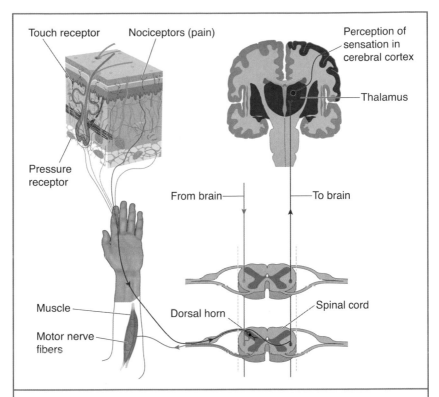

Figure 1.2 This diagram depicts how pain signals are detected and transmitted to the spinal cord and ultimately to the brain. After the sensory fibers make contact with the dorsal horn of the spinal cord, they cross over to the other side before they go up to the brain. Because of this, the left side of the brain receives pain signals from the right side of the body, and vice versa. Different kinds of pain relievers act at different locations in this process to reduce the perception of pain.

THE ANATOMY OF PAIN

Figure 1.2 demonstrates how pain messages are sent to the brain. Pain signals originate in nociceptors located on nerve endings in the skin, muscles, the thin coating of bones, and internal organs. When activated by tissue damage, burns, mechanical disruption, or extreme pressure or temperatures, the nociceptors send signals along the long sensory nerve fibers to the spinal cord. Repeated activation of nociceptors causes them to release inflammatory chemicals called *prostaglandins* (prah-stuh-glan'-dins), which make them extremely sensitive. The sensory nerve fibers that transmit pain signals are divided into two types: *A-delta (A-δ) fibers,* which are insulated with the fatty substance myelin and transmit fast pain signals (at a rate of 2–30 meters per second) for sharp, localized pain; and *C fibers,* which are not insulated with myelin and conduct pain signals at a slower speed (0.5–2 meters per second) for slower, burning pain. Some sensory nerve fibers (such as those that extend from the spinal cord to the toes) are more than a meter long, whereas others (such as those that go from the teeth to the brain stem) are only a few inches long. Sensory nerve fibers enter the spinal cord and connect to the *dorsal horn.* Here, the nerve fibers make connections with other nerve cells called *synapses* onto neurons called *interneurons.* These then relay the information to other neurons up to the brain. The pain signals enter a region of the brain called the *thalamus,* which is a relay station for all sensory information that comes into the brain. From there, signals are transmitted to the *cerebral cortex,* where the information is perceived and processed on a conscious level, allowing the person to react to the pain.

REACTING TO PAIN WITHOUT THINKING

Even though all pain signals are transmitted to the brain, not all of our responses to pain are carefully thought out. Some responses occur right in the spinal cord, bypassing the brain's input completely. The human body has developed this remarkable ability to react to pain without even thinking, probably because certain types of injuries require such an immediate response that waiting for pain signals to be processed and interpreted by the cerebral cortex would result in too much tissue damage before the appropriate response command could be given.

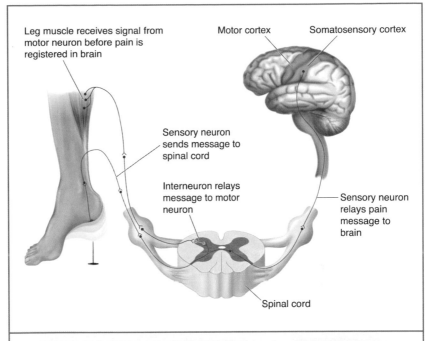

Leg muscle receives signal from motor neuron before pain is registered in brain

Motor cortex

Somatosensory cortex

Sensory neuron sends message to spinal cord

Interneuron relays message to motor neuron

Sensory neuron relays pain message to brain

Spinal cord

Figure 1.3 This diagram illustrates the pain withdrawal reflex. Note how, once the nerve fibers get inside the spinal cord, they split into one branch that goes up to the brain and another branch that goes to the leg muscles to initiate a response before the signals even reach the brain.

This "reacting without thinking" is accomplished through the *pain withdrawal reflex* (Figure 1.3). In this reflex, a sharp, painful stimulus such as stepping on a nail activates nociceptors in the foot and sends pain signals to the spinal cord via fast-acting A-δ sensory neurons. These fibers make synapses (connections) with interneurons in the dorsal horn of the spinal cord. The short interneurons then form a synapse with another neuron, which splits the pain impulse into two separate signals. One branch crosses over to the other side of the spinal cord and relays the signal to the brain by way of the thalamus (not shown in Figure 1.3) and then the cerebral cortex, primarily the *somatosensory cortex*, where all sensory information is first processed. The other branch forms a *motor neuron* (a nerve fiber that controls movement) that extends into the muscles in the leg, signaling them to contract and withdraw the foot from the nail immediately. Both of these signals (one to the brain, the other to the muscles in the leg) are transmitted simultaneously, so the foot is actually withdrawn from the painful stimulus before the brain has time to register and process the pain. So, the next time you touch a hot stove or step barefoot onto something very sharp, you are actually perceiving the pain sensations several fractions of a second *after* your body has already reacted!

2

Over-the-Counter Pain Relievers

Over-the-counter (OTC) pain relievers are sold without a doctor's prescription and can be found at local pharmacies, grocery stores, and mini-marts. They are not nearly as potent as prescription pain relievers such as morphine and Demerol® (see Chapter 3), so they are most often used to treat mild to moderate pain. OTC pain relievers are not as addictive as prescription pain relievers. Nonetheless, there are several side effects of OTC pain relievers that can be serious.

The body produces its own arsenal of molecules that help fight pain and inflammation. The most effective of these are steroids such as cortisone or hydrocortisone (see Chapter 5). However, when we take synthetic versions of these steroids to treat pain, especially if we take them repeatedly over a long period of time, they can have serious health consequences such as skin and tissue damage as well as bone density problems. Fortunately, beginning with the discovery of aspirin, pharmaceutical companies have developed a class of drugs called *nonsteroidal anti-inflammatory drugs* (NSAIDs). These drugs, which make up the majority of OTC pain relievers, are not chemically classified as steroid molecules and do not cause the tissue damage that steroids do. Yet NSAIDs are very good at reducing pain and inflammation. They act primarily by decreasing the formation of lipid (fat) molecules called *prostaglandins* at the site of injury or damage. They accomplish this by inhibiting the activity of an enzyme called *cyclooxygenase* (sy"-klow-ox'-i-jen-ayz, often abbreviated COX). Inhibition of the COX enzyme results in fewer prostaglandin molecules being formed at the site of injury or damage, which, in turn, reduces inflammation. Since prostaglandins stimulate nociceptors on nerve terminals, lowered prostaglandin production means that fewer pain signals are sent to the spinal cord and ultimately to the brain (Figure 2.1), which results in less pain.

When skin or tissue is injured, the damaged cells release various substances, including peptide and lipid (fat) molecules. Some of these lipids get converted into prostaglandins by the COX enzyme, and these prostaglandins then activate nociceptors on nerve endings to send pain signals to the brain. Like NSAIDs, acetaminophen also inhibits COX, but does so only inside the central nervous system, reducing fever and raising tolerance for pain. If the site of injury or damage becomes infected, immune cells migrate to it and release a substance called *histamine*, which also activates nociceptors.

However, the pathway of pain signals arising from tissue and then traveling to the spinal cord and brain is not a one-way street. It turns out that nerve endings in the skin or tissue can also release peptides such as *substance P*, which can alter the activity of immune cells or cause blood vessels to dilate. This causes swelling or further alters the pain response. Thus, not only does damaged tissue communicate with the central nervous system, but the central nervous system also sends chemical feedback to the site of injury or tissue damage.

The prostaglandins produced by the COX enzyme have uses in the body in addition to their role in pain response, including maintaining the health of the stomach lining, regulating blood flow to the kidneys, and enabling specialized blood cells called *platelets* to initiate the process of blood clotting. Because the COX enzyme is responsible for all of these other functions, there are some potentially harmful side effects of NSAIDs, as will be discussed below.

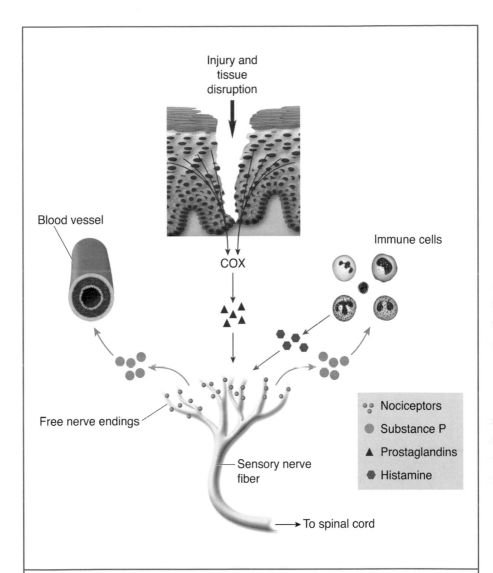

Figure 2.1 This figure illustrates the main chemical messengers involved in producing pain signals. Injured tissue cells release lipids that are converted into prostaglandins by the COX enzyme, which then activate nociceptors on sensory nerve fibers. Immune cells at the site of damage can release histamine, which also activates nociceptors. Nerve endings can also release peptides such as substance P, which alter the activity of immune cells or make blood vessels dilate and cause swelling.

ASPIRIN

Aspirin (Figure 2.2), also known as acetylsalicylic acid (often abbreviated ASA), is one of the oldest OTC pain relievers (see the box on page 28 for aspirin's history). An estimated 30 billion aspirin tablets are consumed every year worldwide. Aspirin is considered an NSAID and inhibits the function of the COX enzyme in producing prostaglandins (see Figure 2.1). Aspirin is also an excellent *antipyretic* (fever reducer), because it promotes the dilation of blood vessels, which cools the skin. In the United States, aspirin is sold under common brand names such as Acuprin®, ASA, Ascriptin®, Aspergum®, Bayer®, Bufferin®, Buffinol, Cope, Doan's®, Ecotrin®, Empirin®, Halfprin®, Healthprin®, Sloprin, St. Joseph®, and ZORprin.

Aspirin takes approximately 30 minutes to start working after you take it by mouth. When taken on a full stomach, it may take longer to work. Aspirin tablets are manufactured to contain anywhere from 80 to 1,000 milligrams (mg) of aspirin each. Maximum pain relief is observed in adults with a dosage of 3,600 to 5,400 mg of aspirin per day, and the ability of aspirin to relieve pain lasts for about 4 to 6 hours.

Aspirin has some beneficial effects when mixed with caffeine, because caffeine increases the pain-relieving and anti-inflammatory effects of aspirin. Brand names of pain relievers that combine aspirin and caffeine include Alka-Seltzer®, Anacin®, and Cope Analgesic Pain Reliever.

Aspirin is considered a relatively safe medication, but it does have some potentially dangerous side effects, especially when taken in amounts that exceed the recommended dosage or when taken for a prolonged period of time (i.e., weeks or months). Such side effects include tinnitus (ringing in the ears), upset stomach and stomach ulcers, liver or kidney problems, and high blood pressure. Aspirin also reduces the blood's ability to form clots; for this reason, aspirin is considered a "blood thinner." This reduced blood clotting can result in bleeding from the stomach or intestines.

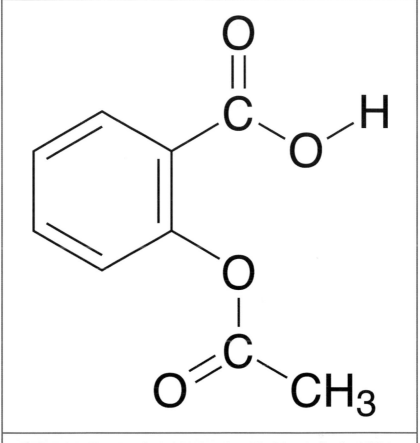

Figure 2.2 The chemical structure of aspirin (acetylsalicylic acid) is shown here.

Although the ability of aspirin to inhibit blood clotting can be dangerous, it can also be beneficial, as in the case of a heart attack. Heart attacks are caused by a blockage of the blood vessels that provide the heart muscle with its own blood supply. This blockage is often caused by blood clots. Since aspirin inhibits the formation of blood clots, it can substantially reduce the risk of the occurrence of a heart attack. Aspirin can even reduce the damage to the heart if it is taken during a heart attack.

A BRIEF HISTORY OF ASPIRIN

200 B.C.   The Greek physician Hippocrates discovers that having his patients chew on bark and leaves from the willow tree (which contains high amounts of a substance called salicin) significantly reduces pain and fever.

A.D. 100–200   The use of willow leaves for the relief of pain is described in the writings of early Roman doctors and Greek surgeons.

1832   A German chemist experiments with salicin and creates salicylic acid.

1897   Another German chemist, Felix Hoffmann, working for the drug company Bayer, synthesizes a stable form of acetylsalicylic acid, which becomes the major active ingredient in aspirin.

1899   Aspirin makes its debut as a pain reliever and is distributed to physicians in powdered form by Bayer. Aspirin is available by prescription only.

1900   Aspirin is distributed in water-soluble tablets, cutting the cost of the medication in half.

1915   Aspirin becomes available without a prescription.

ACETAMINOPHEN

Like aspirin, acetaminophen (Figure 2.3a) inhibits the activity of the COX enzyme and reduces the formation of prostaglandins. However, acetaminophen has the peculiar ability to inhibit only the COX enzymes that are located

1948 A California doctor discovers that approximately 400 of his male patients who take aspirin on a regular basis have no history of heart attack, suggesting that aspirin's ability to reduce blood clotting may somehow prevent the occurrence of heart attacks.

1971 British pharmacologist John R. Vane discovers that aspirin works by reducing the formation of prostaglandins and therefore reducing pain. He is awarded the Nobel Prize for this discovery in 1982.

1980s–1990s The U.S. Food and Drug Administration (FDA) approves the use of aspirin to reduce the risk of stroke and heart attack and recommends that aspirin actually be taken *during* a heart attack to minimize damage to the heart.

1999 Aspirin is inducted into the Natural Museum of American History at the Smithsonian Institute for its century of reducing pains, aches, fevers, and inflammation, and for saving the lives of thousands of heart attack patients.

Source: Bayer. "The History of Aspirin." Available online at *http://www.bayeraspirin.com/press/factsheets/aspirin_history.pdf*.

within the central nervous system (brain and spinal cord) and not the COX enzymes that are located in tissue such as skin and muscle. By acting only on COX enzymes within the central nervous system, acetaminophen actually increases a person's tolerance for pain, although the medical reasons for this are

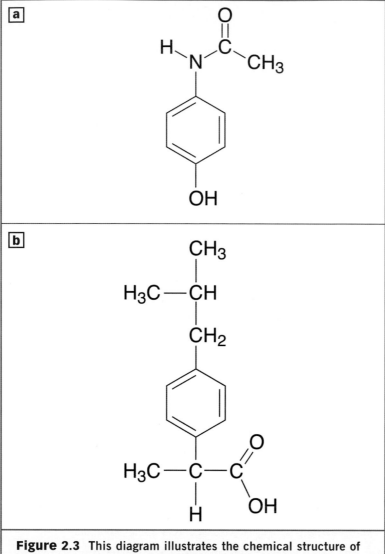

Figure 2.3 This diagram illustrates the chemical structure of acetaminophen (top) and ibuprofen (bottom).

still unknown. Acetaminophen also reduces fever by acting in a region of the brain called the *hypothalamus*, which regulates body heat (among other things). However, acetaminophen does not reduce tissue inflammation and is therefore not considered an NSAID. Common brand names of acetaminophen in the United States are Anacin-3®, Bromo-Seltzer®, Datril®, FeverAll®, Panadol®, and Tylenol®.

Unlike aspirin, acetaminophen does not alter the body's blood-clotting abilities and therefore does not have aspirin's potential benefits in reducing heart attacks and strokes. On the other hand, acetaminophen does not have the toxic side effects of aspirin such as intestinal bleeding and stomach ulcers. However, like most OTC drugs, acetaminophen is metabolized by the liver, and when taken repeatedly in amounts that exceed the recommended dosage, it can cause liver damage.

Acetaminophen comes in tablet and liquid forms that range from 80 to 650 mg per dose. The recommended dosage for adults is approximately 4,000 mg per day. Acetaminophen takes about 30 minutes to start working and lasts approximately 4 to 6 hours. Taking too much acetaminophen can cause nausea, vomiting, and anorexia (loss of appetite).

Acetaminophen can interact with other drugs, both in good and bad ways. For example, hospitals often combine acetaminophen with the narcotic pain reliever codeine (CoTylenol®) to treat more severe pain. Caffeine can increase the effectiveness of acetaminophen similarly to the way it does with aspirin. Brand names that use a combination of aspirin, caffeine, and acetaminophen include Excedrin® and Vanquish®. Combining these ingredients for their additive effects also reduces the dose needed for each one and thereby reduces the risk of side effects. However, there are a few drugs that should not be mixed with acetaminophen. These include anticonvulsants and alcohol, both of which increase the risk of liver damage.

IBUPROFEN

Just like aspirin and acetaminophen, ibuprofen (Figure 2.3b) inhibits the COX enzyme and reduces the formation of prostaglandins. Ibuprofen inhibits COX enzymes both inside

JENNIFER'S SIDE EFFECTS OF IBUPROFEN

Jennifer was a year-round athlete in high school. She ran long-distance races for the track team, was on the cross-country team, and played varsity soccer. During her junior and senior years, she started to have pain in both of her knees, and her doctor diagnosed her with chronic tendonitis, also known as "overuse injury." Jennifer started taking ibuprofen at the maximum recommended dosage—1,200 mg per day (two 200-mg tablets in the morning, afternoon, and evening). She took the pills on an empty stomach with hopes of achieving faster pain relief. After 6 months of taking ibuprofen every day, Jennifer started to have stomach cramps and had a "sick" feeling in her stomach much of the time. Even eating regular food sometimes bothered her stomach. These stomach problems continued to get worse as time went on, and eventually, Jennifer went to see her doctor about them. The doctor gave Jennifer a chalky-tasting phosphate liquid to drink and then had X-ray pictures taken of her stomach (the phosphate drink helps the doctor visualize the stomach during X-ray examinations, which are used most often for looking at harder substances such as bones). The X rays revealed that Jennifer had early signs of stomach ulcers, since the lining of her stomach was starting to erode in several places. Jennifer's blood was drawn and sent to the laboratory, which revealed that she was borderline anemic (had abnormally low blood iron levels). The doctor recommended decreasing the dose and frequency of ibuprofen and also recommended that Jennifer take the medication on a full stomach. He also told her to eat red meat to increase her blood iron level. This was hard to do, since Jennifer was a vegetarian.

Jennifer decided to stop taking ibuprofen altogether, and within 2 to 3 months, her stomachaches had disappeared. However, to this day, Jennifer's stomach is still very sensitive to any medications that contain ibuprofen.

and outside the central nervous system. Therefore, it can reduce inflammation at the site of tissue damage or injury. Ibuprofen is considered an NSAID and also reduces fever. Common brand names of ibuprofen in the United States are Advil®, Cramp End®, Excedrin IB®, Medipren®, Midol®, Motrin®, Motrin IB®, and Nuprin®. Most people tend to tolerate ibuprofen better than aspirin and acetaminophen, and it causes fewer side effects such as intestinal bleeding and stomach ulcers. However, some problems can occur with prolonged and repeated ibuprofen use.

Ibuprofen comes in tablet and liquid forms that range from 50 to 200 mg per dose. Tablets with doses up to 800 mg of ibuprofen are available with a doctor's prescription. The recommended dosage for adults is approximately 1,200 mg per day, but a doctor can suggest that the patient take up to 3,200 mg per day. Ibuprofen is generally well tolerated, but some people can have side effects such as stomach pains, skin rash, vomiting, black or darkened stools, visual problems, or swelling of the hands and feet. Like aspirin and acetaminophen, ibuprofen takes about 30 minutes to start to relieve pain and lasts approximately 4 to 6 hours.

Ibuprofen should not be combined with acetaminophen or other anti-inflammatory medications, because of the possibility of toxic effects on the liver and kidneys. In addition, repeatedly taking ibuprofen in combination with alcohol may cause stomach ulcers or bleeding.

NAPROXEN

Naproxen is a chemical cousin of ibuprofen. Both are derived from a chemical called propionic acid. Common brand names of naproxen in the United States are Aleve®, Anaprox®, Naprelan®, and Naprosyn®. Like ibuprofen, naproxen is an NSAID that inhibits the COX enzyme and reduces pain, fever, and inflammation. The advantage of using naproxen instead of ibuprofen is that naproxen remains in the blood longer (8–12 hours compared with 4–6 hours for ibuprofen) and does not need to be taken as often. Naproxen comes in tablets or capsules of approximately 220 mg each, although tablets containing higher doses can be obtained with a doctor's prescription. The recommended daily dosage for naproxen ranges from 440 to 1,250 mg per day for adults. Naproxen takes about 30 minutes to start relieving pain.

Despite acting for a longer period of time, naproxen has a slightly greater risk of side effects than ibuprofen. Possible side effects include nausea, heartburn, dizziness, headache, drowsiness, ringing in the ears, stomach pain and ulcers, skin rashes, and swelling of the hands and feet. As with ibuprofen, naproxen should not be combined with acetaminophen or other anti-inflammatory medications, because of possible toxic effects on the liver and kidneys. In addition, repeatedly taking naproxen in combination with alcohol may lead to stomach ulcers or bleeding.

NEWER NSAIDS

Throughout the 1980s and 1990s, scientists succeeded in unraveling the mystery of why NSAIDs were so effective in reducing inflammation and pain while at the same time causing harmful side effects such as upset stomach, ulcers, and intestinal bleeding. It turns out that there are two forms of the COX enzyme that produce prostaglandins: COX-1 and COX-2. COX-1 is involved in the processes of blood clotting and maintaining a healthy stomach lining, whereas COX-2 is primarily responsible for inflammation in the skin and muscle tissue that causes pain. NSAIDs such as aspirin, ibuprofen, and naproxen inhibit the activity of *both* the COX-1 and COX-2 enzymes. This results in pain relief but also toxic side effects.

After recognizing this problem, scientists and pharmaceutical companies aimed to develop NSAIDs that specifically inhibit COX-2 but not COX-1. The rationale was that creating an NSAID that inhibits only COX-2 would reduce the formation of prostaglandins that produce pain and inflammation, but would leave untouched the formation of prostaglandins that regulate blood clotting and stomach lining health.

In 1998, the U.S. Food and Drug Administration (FDA) approved a new drug called celecoxib (Celebrex®) for treatment of rheumatoid arthritis and osteoarthritis. The following year, a drug called rofecoxib (VIOXX®) was approved for treating various types of pain, including menstrual cramps and osteoarthritis. These drugs proved to be effective pain relievers and soon became some of the hottest-selling medications on the market. Recent scientific studies have shown that they may have additional benefits, such as the prevention of certain types of colon cancer. COX-2 inhibitors are still available only by prescription.

Despite being selective COX-2 inhibitors, celecoxib and rofecoxib are not entirely without side effects. Some people have reported that these drugs produce some of the same side effects of other NSAIDs (including nausea, heartburn, swelling of the hands and feet, and skin rashes), especially when taken in combination with other NSAIDs. Side effects are also more common when more than the recommended dosages are taken or the drugs are taken in combination with alcohol. COX-2 inhibitors can also increase blood pressure and cause kidney problems in older adults, and they occasionally cause headaches. There are even some reports that COX-2 inhibitors may actually increase the risk of heart attacks in older adults.

Celecoxib is available in 100- or 200-mg capsules, is long acting, and is not recommended for children. Until recently, rofecoxib (VIOXX) was available in 10- to 50-mg capsules. Although VIOXX has been shown to relieve arthritis pain, Merck, the manufacturer of the drug, voluntarily pulled the drug from the market in September 2004, after new research showed an increased risk of stroke and heart attacks among long-term users.

3

Morphine and Other Opiate Pain Relievers

Among the remedies which it has pleased Almighty God to give to man to relieve his sufferings, none is so universal and so efficacious as opium.
—Thomas Sydenham, 17th-century pioneer of English medicine

NSAIDs only provide relief from mild to moderate pain. When the pain is more severe, such as after major surgery or trauma, the patient may need a type of pain reliever called an *opiate* (oh'-pee-et; sometimes called an opioid), such as morphine, codeine, or Demerol. Opiates are so named because they were originally isolated and extracted from the sap of the opium poppy plant *Papaver somniferum* (Figure 3.1). Opium is also the source of the highly addictive street drug heroin, which, despite its high potential for causing addiction, is an effective pain reliever. Opiates are sometimes called "narcotics" because in high doses they can produce a dazed state of "narcosis," or a dream-like state, resulting from massive reductions in the activity of the nervous system. The ability of opiates to relieve pain has been known for centuries, and they are still used in medicine today as some of the most potent and effective pain relievers.

OPIATE PAIN RELIEVERS

If pain is "moderate," a doctor might consider prescribing an NSAID

(continued on page 40)

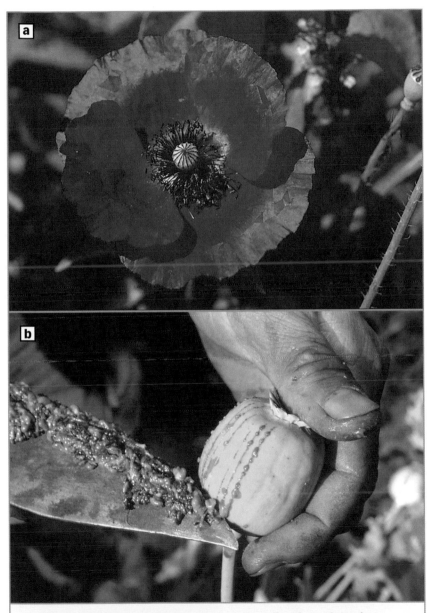

Figure 3.1 Opiate drugs were derived at first from the opium poppy plant, seen here. At top, the plant, whose Latin name is *Papaver somniferum*, is seen in full bloom. In the bottom view, sap is being taken out of the pod for use in making drugs.

A BRIEF HISTORY OF OPIUM

4000 B.C.   Reference to the opium poppy is found in ancient Sumerian texts and Egyptian art.

3200–2600 B.C.   Fossilized opium poppies have been found dating back to Neolithic settlements in what is now Switzerland.

330 B.C.   Alexander the Great, king of Macedonia, introduces opium to Persia and India.

A.D. 400–800   Opium is imported into China, and its use becomes widespread throughout the country.

1729   The smoking and sale of opium in China is made illegal because of the many cases of addiction and overdoses; however, its importation remains legal.

1803   Morphine is extracted and isolated from the sap of the opium poppy by German pharmacist Frederick Serturner. The drug is named after Morpheus, the Greek god of dreams, for its ability to make the user extremely sedated.

1832   Codeine is extracted and isolated from opium.

Mid-1800s   The Opium Wars are fought between China (a leading importer of opium) and Great Britain (a leading exporter of opium) after China bans the drug's importation and use. China is defeated and forced to allow importation of opium from Great Britain.

1850–1865   Waves of Chinese immigrants come to the United States during a labor shortage, bringing opium and opiate addiction with them.

1861–1865   U.S. Civil War soldiers are treated with opium for battle wounds, and many of them become addicted.

1874 In an attempt to provide a nonaddicting alternative to opium and morphine, English pharmacist C. R. Adler boils morphine in acetic acid to produce diacetylmorphine (heroin).

1878 San Francisco, California, passes a city ordinance banning the visitation or patronage of opium houses, although the importation, sale, and possession of opium remains legal.

1887 The United States bans the importation of opium by Chinese immigrants (but not by U.S. citizens).

1898 The Bayer Company sells heroin as a cough suppressant and substitute for morphine. It quickly becomes the best-selling drug of all time.

Early 1900s An estimated 27% of the adult male population (3.5% of the total population) of China is addicted to opium.

1914 The U.S. government passes the Harrison Narcotic Act, which taxes the sale of opiates and prohibits the sale of opiates by certain individuals.

1922 The U.S. government passes the Narcotic Import and Export Act, which prohibits the import and sale of crude opium except for medical purposes.

1924 The U.S. government passes the Heroin Act, making it illegal to manufacture or possess heroin.

1942 The U.S. government passes the Opium Poppy Control Act, banning the growing of opium poppy plants in the United States.

(continued from page 36)

combined with an opiate, such as CoTylenol (codeine + Tylenol). When used in combination, the amount of drug needed can be lowered, and the risk of side effects, including addiction, is reduced. These combination drugs don't always work for severe pain, in which case the doctor may prescribe a stronger opiate drug.

The gold standard of opiate pain relievers is morphine. It was one of the first compounds extracted, isolated, and purified from the opium poppy, and it continues to be one of the most widely used pain relievers today. Morphine and other opiate drugs such as heroin, codeine, oxycodone, and hydrocodone have very similar chemical structures (Figure 3.2). However, other opiates such as fentanyl and meperidine (Demerol) have a slightly different structure (Figure 3.3).

Doctors are most likely to prescribe morphine or other opiates when pain is severe and expected to be short-lasting (a few days to a week), such as after injury or major surgery. This is because short-term use of opiates is less likely to lead to tolerance (loss of potency with repeated use of the drug) and dependence (addiction). However, the problem becomes more complex when the severity of the pain requires the use of pain-relieving medication for more than a few weeks, because this is when tolerance and addiction to opiates tend to develop (see the section on Opiate Addiction on page 48).

Table 3.1 on pages 44–45 lists commonly used opiate pain relievers. All opiates require a doctor's prescription. The medications differ primarily by their duration of action and the dose required to obtain sufficient analgesia.

Even with their outstanding usefulness as pain relievers, opiates have several side effects that can be serious. One of the most common side effects is that they are extremely sedating because they cause an overall depression of nervous system activity. This may significantly impair a person's ability to function at work or to drive a car. Opiates also tend to slow a person's breathing, and a complete stoppage of breathing is

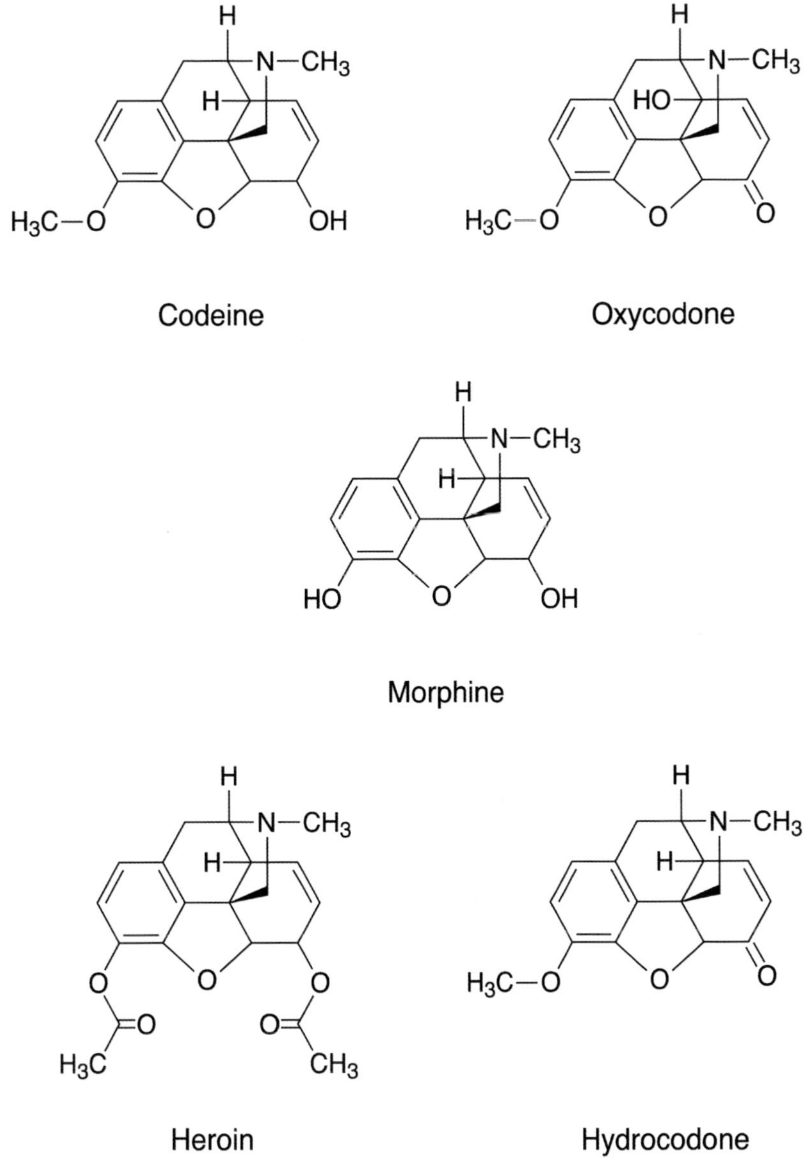

Figure 3.2 This diagram illustrates the chemical structures of morphine, codeine, oxycodone, hydrocodone, and heroin. Notice how each molecule differs from the others by only a few atoms.

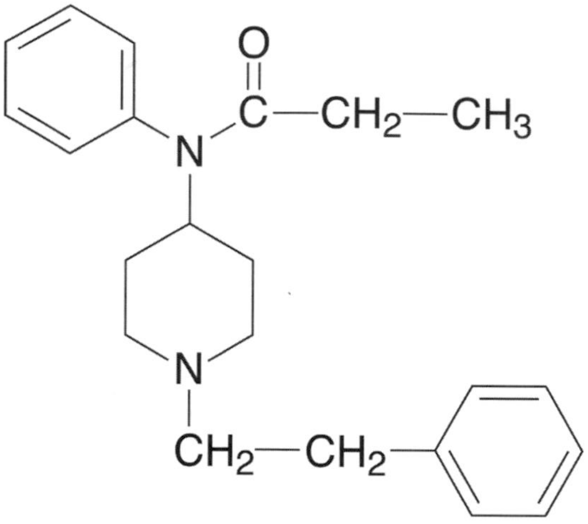

Fentanyl

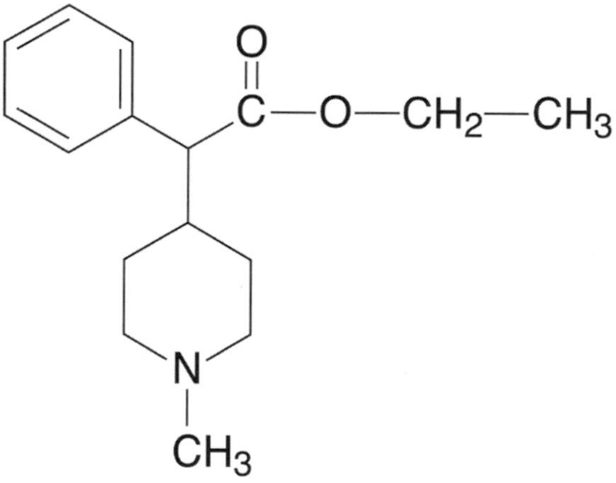

Meperidine

Figure 3.3 These are the chemical structures of fentanyl and meperidine (Demerol).

often the primary reason why opiate overdose results in death. A related problem is that opiates inhibit the cough reflex, which is why opiates are occasionally included in prescription cough medicines. (In fact, heroin was marketed as a cough suppressant in the late 1800s before its addicting properties led the U.S. government to ban it.) Other side effects of opiates are clouded thinking, constipation, dry mouth, nausea, vomiting, lowered blood pressure, sweating, and an inability to urinate. Some opiates induce the release of histamine from immune cells (refer to Chapter 2). This can cause itching and allergic reactions. Finally, tolerance, dependence, and addiction are particularly troubling side effects of opiates.

HOW OPIATES RELIEVE PAIN

Opiate drugs bind to and activate a protein called *mu opiate receptor* (mu is the Greek letter μ; pronounced myoo), which is located on the surface of nerve cells in the dorsal horn of the spinal cord. The dorsal horn is where sensory nerve fibers from the skin, muscle, and internal organs enter the spinal cord before sending their signals to the brain. Activation of the mu opiate receptor by opiate drugs inactivates the nerve cells on which they are located. Thus, pain signals are not sent to the brain. Mu opiate receptors are also found on neurons in various regions of the brain that process pain signals, including the thalamus and cerebral cortex. Scientists believe opiates may inhibit pain perception by acting in the brain as well as in the dorsal horn of the spinal cord. Mu receptors are also located in brain regions that control respiration, which is why opiate drugs cause the breathing to slow down. Finally, mu opiate receptors are also found outside the central nervous system, such as on nerve endings that control the contraction of the intestines. This is why opiates often cause constipation.

(continued on page 48)

Table 3.1 Opiate Pain Relievers

DRUG NAME	BRAND NAME	DOSES	USES/COMMENTS
Codeine	None when used alone	15–60 mg every 4 hours	Often combined with acetaminophen (CoTylenol®, Penaphen®) for moderate pain
Fentanyl	Sublimaze®, Duragesic®	0.01–0.1 mg per hour	30–125 times more potent than morphine; can be given via skin patch; also used as an epidural during childbirth
Hydrocodone	None when used alone	5–10 mg every 4–6 hours	Most often combined with acetaminophen (Anexsia®, Azolone, Damason®, Lorcet®, Lortab®, Vicodin®, Zydone®) or ibuprofen (Vicoprofen®)
Hydromorphone	Dilaudid®, Hydrostat®	2–10 mg every 4–6 hours	5 times more potent than morphine
Meperidine	Demerol	50–100 mg every 3 hours	An effective pain reliever but potentially fatal if given in combination with antidepressants known as MAO (monoamine oxidase) inhibitors; can also cause seizures
Methadone	Dolophine®, Methadose®	5–40 mg; lasts 4–6 hours or longer	Because it is less addictive and stays in the body longer, methadone is often used to wean addicts off heroin or other opiates

DRUG NAME	BRAND NAME	DOSES	USES/COMMENTS
Morphine	Kadian®, MS Contin®, Oramorph®	10–30 mg every 4 hours	More effective when given intravenously than orally; can also be used as an epidural during childbirth
Oxycodone	OxyContin®, Roxicodone®	5 mg every 6 hours	Often combined with aspirin (Percodan®) or acetaminophen (Percocet®, Roxicet, Tylox®); is quickly absorbed into the bloodstream when crushed into a powder; produces profound euphoria and often addiction
Oxymorphone	Numorphan®	1–2 mg every 4–6 hours	Can be used as epidural medication as well as for presurgical sedation
Propoxyphene	Darvon®	50–100 mg every 4 hours	Very weak potency (similar to aspirin); can be combined with acetaminophen (Darvocet®, E-Lor®, Genagesic, Propacet®, Wygesic®)
Tramadol	Ultram®	50 mg every 4–6 hours	Although not chemically related to opiates, it seems to act in a very similar fashion

CONTROLLING YOUR LEVEL OF PAIN

Normally, opiate pain relievers are prescribed to nonhospitalized patients in the form of a pill or tablet, which can take 30 to 60 minutes to start working. If the patient is in the hospital, opiates are usually given intravenously by a doctor or nurse. In this case, whenever the pain-relieving effects of the opiate wear off, the doctor or nurse is summoned to give the patient another dose.

Recent advances in technology have allowed doctors and scientists to develop a method that allows the patient to control the intravenous administration of the pain medication. This technique is called *patient-controlled analgesia* (PCA). With PCA, the pain medication (e.g., codeine or morphine) is dissolved and put into a syringe that is located in a computerized syringe pump. The syringe is connected to plastic tubing and a hypo-dermic needle or catheter that has already been placed into a vein, usually in the patient's wrist or forearm (Figure 3.4). The patient pushes a button on the remote control device of the PCA, and the syringe pump automatically delivers a specific amount of the drug solution into the bloodstream. In this way, whenever the patient begins to feel pain, more pain medication is only a click of the button away.

PCA does not allow the patient to administer too much of the drug. To avoid overdosing, the doctor specifies how much drug is delivered with each dose, and the syringe pump has a "lockout" mechanism—even if the patient continues to press the button, no more of the drug will be delivered for a specific amount of time (usually for 5 to 10 minutes).

The advantage of PCA is that the patient is able to administer the precise amount of pain medication needed to control his or her pain without having to see the doctor every time an injection is needed. This way, the patient can maintain more constant levels of pain medication in the bloodstream. Also, since the pain-relieving effects and side effects of

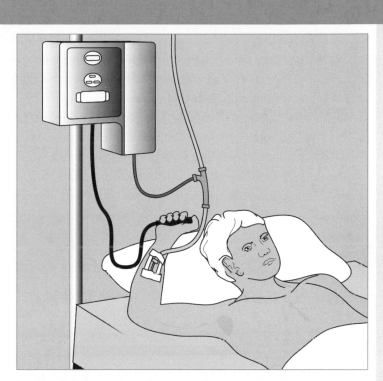

Figure 3.4 *Patient-controlled analgesia, or PCA (illustrated here) allows a patient to control his or her own dosing of a pain relieving medication—to an extent. When the patient presses a button, the drug is delivered through an intravenous (IV) needle. The doctor can decide how much of the drug should be delivered in each dose and how many doses a patient may have within a prescribed time period. The device will lock after that limit is reached, preventing the patient from overdosing.*

different opiates can vary widely from one pain patient to another, PCA allows the patient to inject more or less of drug, depending upon his or her individual needs. Finally, many pain patients, particularly those who have cancer, find that having an influence over their own pain relief gives them greater peace of mind and a sense of control over their own suffering.

(continued from page 43)

Our bodies have their own pain-relieving system: They produce substances that activate the mu opiate receptor. These substances, such as endorphins, are known as *endogenous opiates* because they come from within the body. Opiate drugs are known as *exogenous opiates* because they come from outside the body. Under conditions of extreme stress or emotion or even during moderate to heavy exercise or physical exertion, nerve cells within the central nervous system release endorphins. These bind to the mu opiate receptor and inhibit our perception of pain. Scientists believe this is why our ability to feel pain is dramatically reduced during extremely stressful or emotional events such as an automobile accident or military combat, or during intense physical activity such as running a marathon.

OPIATE ADDICTION

Addiction to prescription opiate pain relievers is a serious and growing problem in many countries, including the United States. The National Survey on Drug Use and Health revealed that more than 2.5 million people either abused or became addicted to prescription opiate pain relievers in the year 2000. This is up from about 600,000 in 1990 (Figure 3.5). This survey also showed that approximately 30 million people in the United States have abused prescription opiate pain relievers at some point in their lives. Public awareness of the problem has increased thanks to the confessions or exposures of celebrities who have had problems with addiction to pain relievers. Such celebrities include conservative radio talk show host Rush Limbaugh; musicians Elvis Presley, Michael Jackson, Kurt Cobain, Courtney Love, and James Brown; television personalities Ozzy, Jack, and Kelly Osbourne (*The Osbournes*) and Matthew Perry (*Friends*); movie stars Winona Ryder, Elizabeth Taylor, and Chris Farley; and even professional sports icons such as National Football League (NFL) quarterback Brett Favre. The wide range of people who have struggled with drug addiction shows that everyone is vulnerable to becoming addicted to opiates.

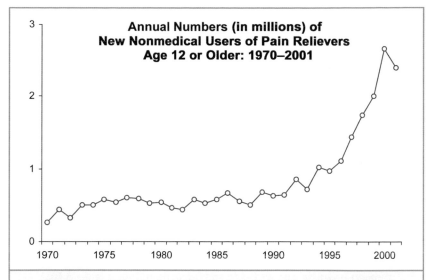

Figure 3.5 This graph depicts the numbers of people (in millions) who starting abusing or became addicted to prescription pain relievers between 1970 and 2001.

Addiction and abuse of narcotic pain relievers are often referred to as "nonmedical use," because the user no longer takes the medication for pain relief, but for another reason such as the *euphoria* (intensely pleasurable feelings, often called a "high") that the drugs produce. This euphoria is not normally experienced when drugs like OxyContin are taken orally as they are supposed to be, because the drug is absorbed slowly in the stomach and into the bloodstream over a period of several hours. However, people have discovered that by crushing the OxyContin pills into a fine powder and then snorting the powder or injecting it intravenously, they can get a quick and intense high. Reports of this new way to get high spread quickly over the Internet, and soon OxyContin became a popular drug sold on the street. However, the government and pharmaceutical industries soon began to take steps to counter the fast rise in prescription pain reliever abuse. Such measures included discontinuing the sale of the higher dosage

(continued on page 52)

EPIDURAL ADMINISTRATION OF OPIATES

Side effects such as sedation, slowed breathing, and reduced blood pressure often result when opiates are given by mouth or by injection. However, in certain situations, such as during childbirth, the patient needs to be alert and responsive and to have proper functioning of the respiratory and cardiovascular systems while at the same time being relieved of severe pain. To allow this to occur, physicians often use a technique called *epidural anesthesia.* With the patient lying on his or her side, a needle is carefully inserted between the vertebrae into the region immediately surrounding the spinal cord, called the *epidural space.* Then, a small amount of opiate drug (such as fentanyl or morphine) is injected into the epidural space through a syringe connected to some plastic tubing (Figure 3.6). The opiate drug then binds to mu opiate receptors in the dorsal horn of the spinal cord and inhibits the activity of nerve cells that transmit pain signals to the brain. The injection is usually made in the lower back region where nerve fibers from the pelvic area enter the spinal cord. Because the drug remains confined to this small, localized area within the spinal cord, the patient feels no pain in the pelvic region, yet remains awake, alert, and responsive. When the drug is administered into the epidural space, it does not flow to the rest of the body, so the patient does not experience other side effects of opiates such as nausea and vomiting. Finally, because less of the drug is needed during an epidural than for oral or intravenous administration, it takes less time for the drug to be eliminated from the body. The result is a quicker recovery time.

There are, however, some side effects of epidural anesthesia. The patient's legs often become numb, and movement of the leg muscles is difficult. Other mild side effects include a backache (thought to be a result of over-relaxation of the back muscles), itchiness of the skin, and an inability to urinate. More rarely, patients experience headache, lowered blood

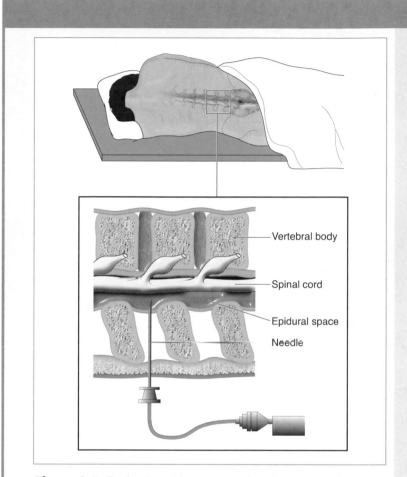

Figure 3.6 *During an epidural, a patient is given a strong anesthetic through an injection into the spinal canal. This allows for pain relief in the lower body (below the point of injection), while the upper body remains unaffected, allowing breathing and heart rate to continue as normal. An epidural is often used to ease the pain of childbirth.*

pressure, bleeding from the point of needle insertion, and patchy numbness (usually in the legs) that can last for up to three months after the epidural.

CHOOSING NOT TO HAVE AN EPIDURAL

During the birth of a baby, the baby's head—which is about 4 to 5 inches in diameter—must squeeze through the birth canal, which normally does not stretch beyond 2 inches in diameter without pain or tearing. In addition, the repeated contractions of the uterus that help to push out the baby are very painful. Nevertheless, some women choose not to receive an epidural during childbirth. Why would a woman decide against relieving what is probably the most excruciating pain a human can experience? Many fear having adverse effects of an epidural, such as headache, itchiness, and lingering numbness. Others fear losing control of the abdominal, leg, and uterine muscles that help push the baby along. Some fear that the drug may spread to the baby's circulatory system and sedate the baby, although this is rare. In many cases, the mere thought of having a needle inserted directly into the spine makes the woman refuse an epideral. Still other women believe that "natural" childbirth (without any pain medication) is the way nature meant childbirth to be.

Regardless of the reason, an epidural is always a pain relief option that is properly left to the patient. Some expectant mothers who have decided not to have an epidural end up changing their minds once labor has begun and is not too far advanced.

(continued from page 49)

form of the pills and issuing warnings to physicians regarding the potential for opiate pain reliever abuse. Also, since growing numbers of pharmacies were being robbed for their supply of OxyContin and other opiates, many pharmacies have required patients to preorder their medications several days in advance so that large quantities of these drugs did not have to be kept on hand.

The risk of becoming addicted to an opiate pain reliever increases the longer the drug is taken (over a period of weeks or

VICODIN ADDICTION—SOMETIMES SUBTLE, SOMETIMES NOT

When 58-year-old Molly was vacationing in Australia, she had a sudden mishap. She was riding in a rental car with her husband behind the wheel when he misinterpreted a traffic signal (a common occurrence in a foreign country) and got broadsided by another car on the passenger side. Molly suffered fractured ribs, a fractured sternum, and a bruised lung (fortunately, she was wearing her seatbelt or her injuries might have been even worse). She was taken to the hospital for observation and treatment for several days and returned home to the United States the day after she was discharged from the hospital. A few days after she arrived home, she visited her doctor to get some medication for her pain. The doctor prescribed Vicodin (5 mg of hydrocodone + 500 mg acetaminophen per dose) to take every 4 to 6 hours. As with many opiates, Vicodin made Molly constipated, and she ate prunes to help offset her intestinal problems. Since broken bones heal slowly, Molly kept taking Vicodin for over a month before switching to an OTC pain reliever. Immediately after she stopped taking Vicodin, however, Molly started to have insomnia. She was only getting 4 to 5 hours of sleep per night. When she was able to sleep, it was very fitful and restless. The sleep problems finally disappeared about a month after she stopped taking Vicodin. Fortunately, insomnia was the only apparent "withdrawal" symptom Molly experienced after stopping Vicodin. Others are not so lucky.

A 25-year-old woman named Doris was also involved in a car accident. The injuries she sustained required her to start taking a regimen of Vicodin similar to what Molly had taken. Before long, Doris's body just couldn't live without the Vicodin and she became addicted to the medication. Her doctor refused to give her any more prescription refills. He felt she was well past the point where she should be having pain from her original injuries. Soon, Doris found herself forging prescriptions for Vicodin—a felony in many states. Eventually, the law caught up with her, and she was arrested and sentenced to jail for prescription forgery. Even after serving time in prison, Doris had to enroll in a court-ordered drug rehabilitation program. Her job and relationships with family and friends all suffered during her struggle with Vicodin addiction.

Although not everyone becomes severely addicted to opiate pain relievers, there are certain people for whom the drugs become irresistible. The addiction may drive these ordinarily upstanding individuals to criminal behavior to satisfy their craving and compulsive need for these medications.

months, as opposed to only a few days). One reason this is true is because when opiate drugs are taken repeatedly, the body starts to react and adapt to the presence of the drug in the body. Eventually, the drug becomes less potent, and the person needs to take more of it to achieve the same effect. This phenomenon is known as *tolerance* and is thought to contribute to the development of all drug addictions, including addiction to pain relievers.

Once a person has taken an opiate pain reliever for a long enough period of time (weeks or months), he or she may be considered *dependent* on, or addicted to, the drug. This dependence can be physiological, psychological, or both. One foolproof way to tell whether a person is dependent on a certain drug is to have him or her stop taking the drug for a few days. If symptoms of *withdrawal* appear (in the case of opiates, these often include sweating, shaking, diarrhea, cold and clammy skin with goosebumps, headache, nausea, vomiting, stomach cramps, runny nose, insomnia, anxiety, confusion, irritability, fever, increased heart and respiration rate, and intense craving for the drug),

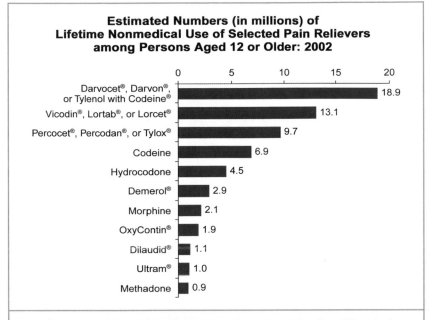

Estimated Numbers (in millions) of Lifetime Nonmedical Use of Selected Pain Relievers among Persons Aged 12 or Older: 2002

Figure 3.7 This graph shows the estimated number (in millions) of people who have used various opiate pain relievers for nonmedical purposes at some point in their lifetime (as of 2002). Considering the dangers of taking opiate drugs for nonmedical reasons, these figures are alarming.

then this is a good sign that the person has developed opiate dependence. Without medical treatment, withdrawal symptoms are most intense for 1 to 2 days after stopping the drug and can last 5 to 7 days. However, under the supervision of a physician, these withdrawal symptoms can be reduced with other medications.

As seen in Figure 3.7, the most widely abused opiate pain relievers are Darvocet®, Darvon®, and Tylenol with codeine®, followed by Vicodin, Lortab®, and Lorcet®. Methadone is the least addicting of the opiate pain relievers and stays in the body the longest. Because of this, methadone is often used as a substitute for morphine, heroin, and other more addictive opiates to "wean" people off the drug to which they are addicted.

4

Antidepressants, Anticonvulsants, Muscle Relaxants, and Migraine Medications

Opioids, NSAIDs, acetaminophen, and COX-2 inhibitors (all discussed in previous chapters) are the most commonly used pain relievers, but they do not relieve all types of pain. *Neuropathic pain* (also called *neuropathy*) and migraine headaches are for the most part unaffected by these pain relievers, so different medications are used to treat these conditions.

Neuropathic pain results from damage to nerve fibers caused by viruses, toxins, physical injury, or diseases such as multiple sclerosis, shingles, and diabetes. When nerve fibers become damaged, they constantly send pain signals to the brain. This results in a state of chronic pain. It is surprising that medications originally designed to treat other disorders (such as depression and epilepsy) are actually effective in alleviating neuropathic pain. Such medications include antidepressants, anticonvulsants, and muscle relaxants. Other specially designed medications to treat migraine headaches (discussed later in this chapter) have also been developed. All these medications are available only by prescription.

ANTIDEPRESSANTS

When nerve cells communicate with each other, they release chemical messengers called neurotransmitters. Two of these are *norepinephrine* (also called *noradrenaline*) and *serotonin*. Both norepinephrine and serotonin regulate mood and emotion. Normally, when a nerve signal ends, these chemical messengers are absorbed back into the nerve cells from which they were released. There, they can be recycled for sending future signals. This process is known as *reabsorption* or *reuptake*. Scientists believe that somewhere in the brains of people who suffer from depression, nerve cells release abnormally low levels of norepinephrine and/or serotonin. Antidepressants block this reabsorption of norepinephrine and/or serotonin back into the nerve cell, thus making their effects on neighboring nerve cells last longer. This causes an overall increase in communication between nerve cells that use these two chemical messengers and, for reasons that are still unknown, helps relieve the symptoms of depression.

Surprisingly, antidepressants are also effective in reducing neuropathic pain. We do not know precisely how antidepressants accomplish this, but scientists believe that the increased levels of norepinephrine and/or serotonin outside the nerve cells somehow dampen pain signals that enter the brain from the spinal cord.

Antidepressants generally fall into one of three categories: (1) tricyclic antidepressants (TCAs), which are so named because of their three-ring chemical structure; (2) selective serotonin reuptake inhibitors (SSRIs), which block only the reabsorption of serotonin and not of norepinephrine; and (3) monoamine oxidase (MAO) inhibitors, which inhibit the metabolic breakdown of norepinephrine and/or serotonin.

TCAs appear to be the most effective antidepressants in relieving the symptoms of neuropathic pain. Listed below are some commonly prescribed TCAs with their brand names in parentheses:

- amitriptyline (Elavil®, Endep®)

- amoxapine (Asendin®)

- desipramine (Norpramin®)

- doxepin (Sinequan®, Zonalon, Adapin®)

- nortriptyline (Aventyl®, Pamelor®)

- imipramine (Tofranil®)

- trimipramine (Surmontil®)

Amitriptyline is usually the treatment of choice for neuro-pathic pain. Some selective serotonin reuptake inhibitors (SSRIs) such as fluoxetine (Prozac®), paroxetine (Paxil®), sertra-line (Zoloft®), and clomipramine (Anafranil®) can be used, but they don't appear to be as effective as TCAs. The doses for TCAs in treating neuropathic pain are usually lower than those for treating depression, and the drugs usually start to take effect more quickly in relieving pain than they do in relieving depression. It is interesting that people who suffer from chronic pain often experience symptoms of depression, so TCAs can benefit these people by helping to ease not only their pain but also their depressed mood.

Like all drugs, TCAs and other antidepressants have some negative side effects. Most common are drowsiness, dry mouth, constipation, and weight gain. However, the drowsiness associated with TCA use can actually be beneficial for some neuropathic pain patients, particularly those who have trouble sleeping because of their pain. Different TCAs cause varying degrees of side effects for different people, so a person who suffers from neuropathic pain may have to try several different TCAs to find the one that is most effective in relieving his or her pain while producing the fewest unwanted side effects.

ANTICONVULSANTS

Another type of medication originally designed for a disorder unrelated to pain is the *anticonvulsant* class, also called *anti-epileptics*. *Epilepsy* is a neurological disorder characterized by spontaneous seizures and *convulsions*—dramatic muscle spasms that result in uncontrollable body movements and often a loss of consciousness. An epileptic attack is started by a massive "storm" of electrical signals generated somewhere in the brain, which causes consciousness to become cloudy and leads excessive nerve impulses to be sent to skeletal muscles, making them contract uncontrollably. Epileptic attacks can be mild (resulting in only slight dizziness and "staring into space"), moderate (in which only one side or part of the body starts to convulse and shake), or severe (in which the person loses consciousness and falls to the ground, with severe shaking of the arms, legs, and face muscles). Epileptic attacks usually last from several seconds to several minutes.

Epilepsy can be caused by genetic factors, brain trauma or injury, viral infections, and likely additional factors that have not yet been discovered. Some people, who may not even be diagnosed with epilepsy, may experience seizures in response to certain patterns of lights and sounds. More severe cases sometimes require the part of the brain that is believed to be the source of the massive storm of electrical signals to be removed surgically. However, epileptic seizures are usually treated with anticonvulsant medications.

Anticonvulsant medications act by quieting and calming the activity of nerve cells. They do this by limiting a nerve cell's ability to send electrical impulses or by increasing the activity of chemical messengers in the brain that naturally inhibit the activity of nerve cells. Because anticonvulsants act in all regions of the nervous system, they also quiet the impulses sent by damaged nerves to the skin, muscles, and other tissue. Thus, anticonvulsants can be used to treat the chronic pain associated with conditions such as trigeminal neuralgia (see Chapter 1) and the neuropathy that results from diseases such as diabetes or shingles. Listed here are some of the most common anticonvulsants (with brand names in parentheses) used to treat these types of chronic pain:

- carbamazepine (Tegretol®, Atretol®, Carbatrol®, Epitol®)

- clonazepam (Klonopin®)

- gabapentin (Neurontin™)

- lamotrigine (Lamictal®)

- phenytoin (Dilantin®)

- sodium valproate (Depakene®, Depakote®, Depacon®), also called valproic acid

- topiramate (Topamax®)

Other anticonvulsants include barbiturate drugs such as amobarbital (Amytal®), butabarbital (Butisol®), pentobarbital (Nembutal®), phenobarbital (Barbita, Luminal, Solfoton®), secobarbital (Seconol®), and thiopental (Pentothal®). These anticonvulsants are quite sedating and potentially addictive and are thus prescribed less often.

Because anticonvulsants calm the activity of the brain, they often produce unwanted side effects such as drowsiness, sedation, dizziness, confusion, loss of coordination, and slurred speech. Some anticonvulsants can produce other side effects, such as nausea, vomiting, constipation, double vision, and even abnormal hair growth. As with TCAs, people suffering from chronic pain often have to try several different anticonvulsants before they find the one that is most effective in relieving their pain while having the least amount of unwanted side effects.

MUSCLE RELAXANTS

Pain caused by sprained, pulled, injured, or spastic (overactive) muscles can be treated with muscle relaxants. As it turns out, muscle relaxants are also useful for treating chronic pain caused by diseases such as fibromyalgia (see Chapter 1). Most muscle relaxants block the signal that nerve fibers in the spinal cord send out to skeletal muscles in the arms, legs, back, and other body parts. Some muscle relaxants, however, such as dantrolene, act directly on the muscle itself to reduce contractions, whereas others act at unknown sites within the central nervous system. Here are some common muscle relaxants (with brand names in parentheses) that are used to treat chronic muscle pain:

- baclofen (Lioresal®)

- benzodiazepine drugs (Klonopin®, Valium®)

- carisoprodol (Soma)

- chlorzoxazone (Paraflex®, Parfon®, Remular®)

- cyclobenzaprine (Flexeril®)

- dantrolene (Dantrium®)

- doxacurium (Nuromax®)

- metaxolone (Skelaxin®)

- methocarbamol (Robaxin®)

- pancuronium (Pavulon®)

- pipecuronium (Arduan®)

- rocuronium (Zemuron)

- tizanidine (Zanaflex®)

- vecuronium (Norcuron®)

Because these drugs relax muscles, they can cause prolonged muscle weakness and motor coordination problems. Some of these drugs also act on the central nervous system and cause side effects such as confusion, dizziness, sedation, nausea, and dry mouth. Most muscle relaxants are prescribed for short-term use, since the potential dangers of long-term use are not yet known. Addiction to most muscle relaxants is fairly uncommon, with the exception of benzodiazepines such as Valium.

Finally, it turns out that nature has provided us with an effective muscle relaxant from a most unusual source. *Clostridium botulinum* (Figure 4.1), also known as botulinum toxin or BoTox®, is a type of bacteria that causes a severe and often fatal form of food poisoning. However, this strain of bacteria actually produces a chemical that relaxes muscles and keeps them from contracting. Originally, BoTox was approved by the U.S. Food and Drug Administration for treating cross-eye in children (a condition known as *strabismus*). Injections of BoTox into the muscles that control the movement of the eyes caused these muscles to relax and allowed doctors to "straighten out" the alignment of the eyes. More recently, BoTox has been approved for certain types of cosmetic surgery, to treat the muscle stiffness of cerebral palsy, and now to treat chronic headaches in pain clinics. BoTox can only be given by a licensed physician and must be injected with a syringe locally into the affected muscle (known as an intramuscular injection). BoTox cannot be given orally in the form of a pill.

MIGRAINE MEDICATIONS

Most of us have had or know about "tension" headaches. However, a subset of people suffer from a severe form or recurring headache known as migraine. Migraines are characterized by severe throbbing pain in specific areas of the head such as the temples, eyes, or back of the head. If you've never experienced a migraine, the "brain freeze" that can happen after rapidly eating ice cream or flavored crushed ice almost matches the intensity of a migraine, but lasts only a few seconds, compared with the hours or days that a migraine lasts. Nausea, vomiting, and sensitivity to light often accompany

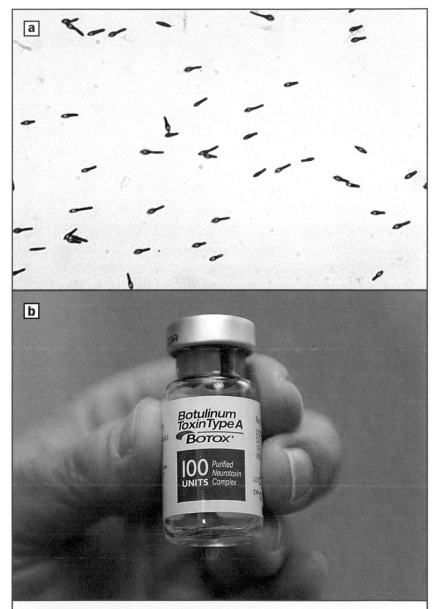

Figure 4.1 At top, *Clostridium botulinum* is seen under a microscope, and at bottom is a vial of BoTox for intramuscular injection. BoTox has become a popular alternative to cosmetic surgery for removing wrinkles.

migraines. In some sufferers of migraine attacks, an aura (seeing flashes of lights and colors or wavy lines) often occurs immediately prior to the headache itself. Migraines can last for several hours or up to a day or longer. Common triggers include changes in weather or air pressure, bright or fluorescent lights or glare, chemical fumes, menstrual cycles, and certain foods such as red or fatty meats, cheeses, red wine, beer, and the food additive monosodium glutamate (MSG). Migraines tend to be more common in males during childhood and in females during adulthood.

WHAT CAUSES MIGRAINES?

Scientists and physicians have pondered for centuries what causes migraine headaches. In the age of Hippocrates, early physicians thought that excess yellow or black bile (fluids the ancient Greeks believed existed in the body) might be to blame. Today, most medical experts believe (though not everyone agrees) that migraines are a result of abnormally low serotonin levels being emitted from the trigeminal nerve (a large nerve that connects to most of the head, including the surface of the brain and its blood vessels). Normally, the blood vessels around the brain are constricted to a certain extent. In migraine sufferers, because the trigeminal nerve gives off little serotonin, the blood vessels can suddenly dilate (widen) and/or become inflamed. This results in the excruciating pain of a migraine headache. Other scientists believe a peptide, made from an enzyme called angiotensin-converting enzyme (ACE) and released by the trigeminal nerve onto blood vessels in the head may also be involved. Drugs that block the action of this peptide are being studied for use as antimigraine medications. In the meantime, a lot of effort is being focused on developing medications that specifically target the serotonin receptors located on the cerebral blood vessels that control their constriction and dilation.

In ancient times, "healers" carved circles out of portions of the skull to attempt to relieve migraines, or they used primitive medications like opium or hemlock extracts. Today, there are more scientifically based medications to treat migraines. These medications can be divided into those that help prevent migraines from recurring (called *preventive* or *prophylactic* treatments) and those that ease the pain or duration of a migraine after it has begun (sometimes called *attack-abortive* treatments).

Preventive Treatments

- **Antidepressants,** such as fluoxetine (Prozac), sertraline (Zoloft), paroxetine (Paxil), venlafaxine (Effexor®), citalopram (Celexa™), as well as certain TCAs, block the reabsorption of serotonin back into nerve cells, which causes excess serotonin to gather around nerve endings. This is believed to cause the blood vessels surrounding the brain to constrict (see Figure 4.2), which helps relieve migraine pain.

- **Beta blockers,** such as propranolol (Inderal®, Lopressor®) and atenolol (Tenormin®), inhibit the actions of norepinephrine on nerve cells. Scientists do not know how these medications relieve migraine symptoms. Beta blockers are also used for the treatment of high blood pressure and chest pain.

- **Calcium channel blockers,** such as verapamil (Calan®, Covera®, Isoptin®, Verelan), diltiazem (Cardizem®, Dilacor®, Tiazac®), and nimodipine (Nimotop®), inhibit the flow of calcium ions into the cells that line blood vessel walls. This changes the way the blood vessels surrounding the brain dilate and constrict and provides relief from migraines.

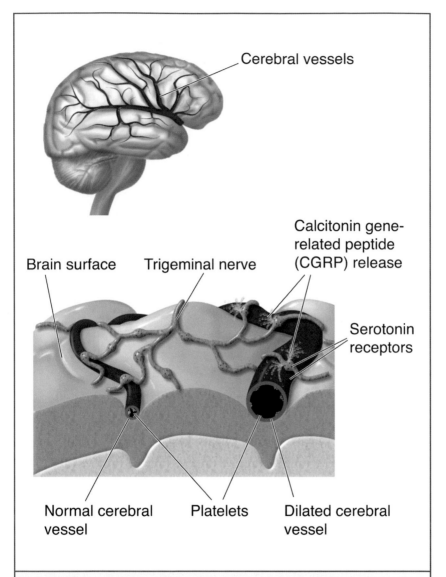

Figure 4.2 Although doctors and scientists are not certain about the cause of migraines, many believe they are a result of changes in the release of chemical messengers (such as serotonin or CGRP) from the trigeminal nerve onto cerebral vessels on the surface of the brain. The result is altered platelet function and/or dilation of the cerebral vessels (illustrated here), which somehow produces the symptoms of migraines.

- **Divalproex sodium (Depakote®)** is used to treat epilepsy and inhibits the firing of nerve cells. This medication appears to be a promising treatment for migraines, although its precise mechanism of action is unknown.

- **Methysergide (Sansert™)** is believed to alter the ability of scrotonin to cause inflammation, platelet aggregation (blood clotting), and dilation of blood vessels. However, methysergide has some undesirable side effects, such as motor incoordination and dizziness and can cause heart problems. Usually, the drug is intentionally discontinued for 4–6 weeks twice a year because of these problems. Thus, methysergide is used only in special cases.

ANDREW'S MIGRAINES

Andrew began to suffer from migraines when he was 6 years old. They came on out of the blue, without any aura, about once a month. The pain was excruciating and mostly localized just behind his eyes. When a migraine attack started, Andrew immediately had to go into a dark room to avoid any additional pain from too much room light and stay there for hours. "It was awful," he recalls. After about 4 to 5 hours of enduring this nightmare, Andrew would feel an overwhelming urge to vomit. After he did so, the migraine would disappear almost immediately. Andrew never took any medications for his migraines.

Andrew was more fortunate than most migraine sufferers. Although migraines do tend to decrease in frequency and intensity when people reach their forties or fifties, Andrew's migraines stopped by the time he graduated from high school. Today, Andrew is a lawyer and has not experienced a migraine in over 10 years.

Attack-Abortive Treatments

- **Ergotamines,** such as Ergomar®, Ergostat®, Cefergot, and DHE 45 (Migranal®) cause the constriction of blood vessels and stimulate the actions of serotonin. Migranal comes as a nasal spray for quick delivery during a migraine attack. However, ergotamines can have undesirable side effects that can even mimic some of the symptoms of migraine itself, such as headache, nausea, and vomiting.

- **Excedrin Migraine** was the first migraine medication to be sold over the counter. It consists of acetaminophen, aspirin, and caffeine.

- **Midrin®** is mixture of a mild blood vessel constrictor called isometheptene mucate, a mild sedative called dichloralphenazone, and acetaminophen. It is mostly used to treat mild migraines. Only mild dizziness and skin rash have been reported as side effects.

- **Opiate narcotics** are used to treat migraines only in extreme cases because of their addictive potential. They also appear to be less effective than some of the other attack-abortive migraine treatments, and they take longer to start working.

- **Triptans,** such as almotriptan (Axert®), electripan (Relpax®), frovatriptan (Frova®), naratriptan (Amerge®), rizatriptan (Maxalt®), sumatriptan (Imitrex®), and zolmitriptan (Zomig®) also cause the blood vessels in the head to constrict and can reduce blood vessel inflammation. The triptans are more widely prescribed than the ergotamines because they have fewer side effects. However, some patients who take triptans experience tingling in the fingers, tightness in the throat, and a bad taste in the mouth. Although some triptans take longer than others to start to relieve the symptoms of migraines, they can be more effective in preventing migraines from recurring. Many triptans come in a nasal spray or "melt-away" pill format that can be taken without water in the event of a sudden migraine attack.

5

Local Anesthetics and Steroids

THE "CAINE" FAMILY OF LOCAL ANESTHETICS

Getting a cavity filled, fixing an ingrown toenail, and having arthroscopic knee surgery are all examples of times when traditional pain relievers in the form of a pill are not the medication of choice. Occasionally, doctors have to treat pain with local anesthetics directly at its source—the nerve fiber endings in the skin, muscle, gums, or teeth, for example. When injected just below the surface of the skin or gums, these anesthetics temporarily inactivate all nerve fibers (not just the nerve fibers that transmit pain sensations but also those that send normal touch sensations). The result is a complete loss of the person's ability to sense pain, touch, or temperature in the specific region of the body where the drug was injected. Sometimes, local anesthetics are used as "nerve block" agents. In such cases, they are injected directly into the region around a damaged nerve in order to stop the repeated pain signals that the nerve is sending. Other nerve blocks are designed to inhibit pain signals from a specific region of the body (such as the jaw or legs) that are carried by a specific nerve. Local anesthetics are also injected directly into the spinal cord as is done in the epidural injection that eases a pregnant woman's pain during childbirth. The advantage of using local anesthetics is that their effects are very temporary and wear off in a relatively short amount of time. A disadvantage of some local anesthetics is that they sometimes diffuse into the bloodstream and have unwanted effects on another part of the body.

The most popular and widely used local anesthetics are those of the "caine" family, so called because their names all end with the suffix "-caine." They are all chemically related to one another (see Figure 5.1 for examples). Some of the more common members of this family (with brand names in parentheses) include:

- **benzocaine** (Americaine®, Hurricaine®, Lanacane®, Anbesol®, Orabase®, Orajel®, Otocain®, Solarcaine®)—Used for relief of pain from sunburn or other skin irritations, ear infections, gum irritations, and dental procedures. Starts to work within 5 to 10 minutes of application and lasts 15 to 45 minutes.

- **bupivacaine** (Anawin, Marcaine®, Sensorcaine®)—Used as a nerve block agent, but not as an epidural during childbirth because it can get into the mother's bloodstream and then enter the bloodstream of the fetus. It takes anywhere from 2 to 30 minutes after administration to take effect, and lasts anywhere from 75 minutes to 6 hours, depending on how it is administered.

- **cocaine**—Despite being one of the most addictive drugs around, cocaine is still used medically as a local anesthetic for surgical procedures on mucous membranes of the mouth, throat, and nose, as well as for some eye surgeries. Peak effects occur in 1 to 5 minutes of application and last 30 minutes or longer.

- **dibucaine** (Nupercainal®)—Used primarily as a topical anesthetic for skin and rectal irritations. It has a slow onset of action because it must penetrate the skin and lasts 30 to 60 minutes.

- **lepobupivacaine** (Chirocaine®)—Used primarily as a long-lasting nerve block agent. It takes up to 15 minutes to have an effect and can last up to 20 hours.

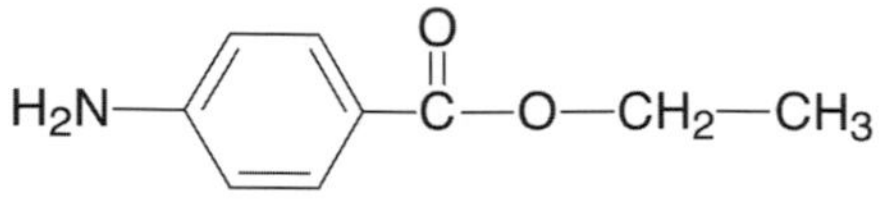

Benzocaine

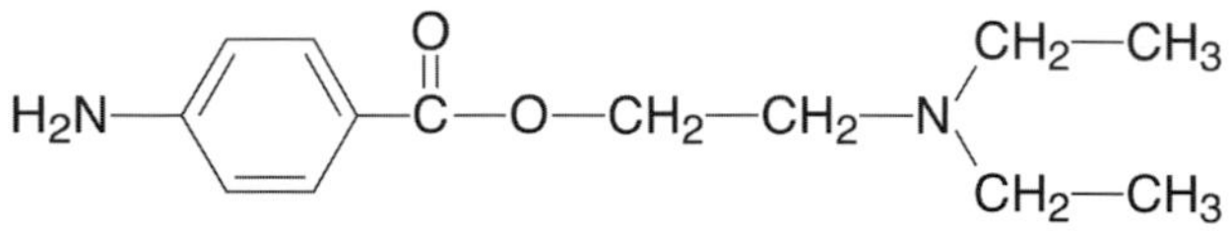

Procaine (Novocaine)

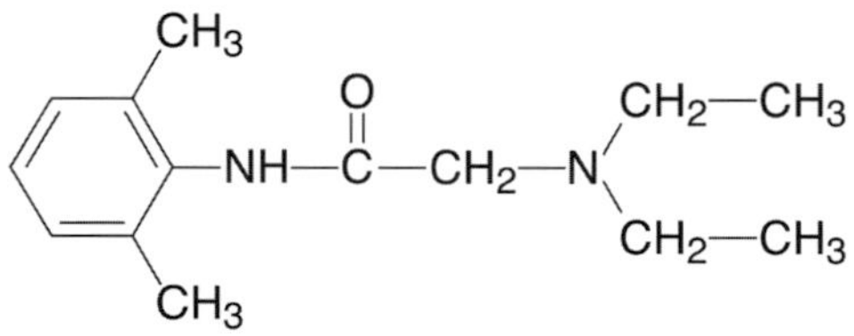

Lidocaine

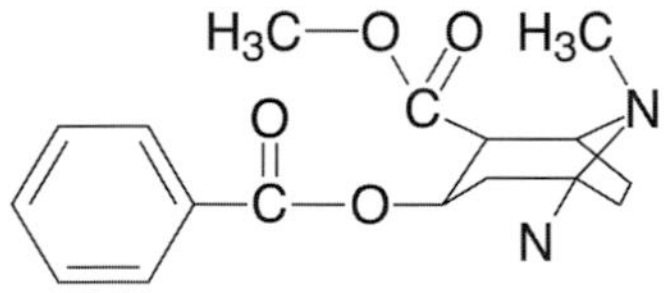

Cocaine

Figure 5.1 Illustrated here are the chemical structures of four common anesthetics. Note how similar they are.

- **lidocaine** (Anestacon®, Dilocaine, L-Caine, Lidoderm®, Lidoject, Nervocaine, Xylocaine®, Zilactin)—A widely used local anesthetic that often comes in a topical ointment and skin patch. Used for providing pain relief from skin irritations and burns, dental surgery, urethral examinations and procedures, and shingles. The onset and duration of action of lidocaine vary according to whether it is applied as an ointment, skin patch, or injection, but normally it takes effect within 15 minutes and lasts for 2 or more hours.

- **mepivacaine** (Carbocaine®, Polocaine®)—Used as a nerve block agent as well as a local anesthetic for dental procedures. It takes effect within 5 minutes and lasts anywhere from 10 minutes to 2 hours.

- **prilocaine** (Citanest®)—Used as a topical anesthetic but also a nerve block agent. It takes effect within 15 minutes and lasts 30 to 90 minutes.

- **procaine** (Novocain®)—One of the most common local anesthetics for dental procedures, it is also used as a nerve block agent. It usually starts to take effect within 5 minutes after administration and lasts up to 1 hour.

- **proparacaine** (Ak-Taine®, Alcaine®, Ophthaine®, Ophthetic®)—Commonly used for eye surgeries. It takes effect within 20 seconds of application and lasts for 15 to 20 minutes.

- **ropivacaine** (Naropin®)—Used for epidurals during normal childbirth as well as caesarean section, but also given as a nerve block agents for postsurgical pain. Takes effects within minutes and lasts up to 6 hours. However, ropivacaine can enter the bloodstream and affect the fetus, so it must be used with caution as an epidural.

- **tetracaine** (Pontocaine®)—Used in eye surgeries and an epidural during childbirth. Also used as a nerve block agent and a local anesthetic on the larynx, trachea, or esophagus. It takes up to 15 minutes to take effect and lasts for up to 3 or 4 hours.

You should keep in mind that the duration of action of most of these local anesthetics can be greatly prolonged if they are taken together with the stimulant epinephrine.

STEROIDS

There are many types of steroid hormones in the body, such as the sex/gonadal hormones testosterone and estrogen, thyroid hormones, growth hormones, and stress hormones, which serve various normal functions. One type of steroid—*corticosteroids* or *glucocorticoids*—is secreted by the adrenal glands (located just above the kidneys). These steroids, particularly synthetic versions of them, have powerful anti-inflammatory actions that help to relieve pain. They are often given as an epidural injection to relieve neck or back pain that results from a compressed or pinched nerve. They can also be injected directly into a joint to relieve pain caused by inflammation in conditions such as tendonitis (inflammation of the tendons), carpal tunnel syndrome, "tennis elbow," bursitis (inflammation of sac-like cavities in tendons or muscles that allow them to slide easily over bone), or other joint pain. Professional athletes, who routinely experience one or more of these conditions, are often given local steroid injections. Frequently, the steroid is combined with a local anesthetic such as lidocaine.

Corticosteroids usually take 3 to 7 days to start to relieve pain, and they are usually injected repeatedly to speed up the process. Prolonged used of corticosteroids to relieve pain can interfere with normal healing processes, weaken tendons, cause bone density problems, and can even damage joint cartilage. Therefore, steroid injections must be used with caution and always under the supervision of a physician.

Some common synthetic corticosteroids used to reduce inflammation (with their brand names in parentheses) are:

- **cortisone** (Cortone®)—In addition to being used to locally treat joint, muscle, or tendon inflammation, cortisone can be used to treat bone pain related to cancer, neuropathic pain, or even headache pain. Its half-life (the time it takes the body to metabolize and excrete half of the amount injected) is 8 to 12 hours.

- **dexamethasone** (Dalalone®, Decadrol, Decadron®, Decaject, Dexasone®, Dexone®, Hexadrol®, Solurex)—Like cortisone, it can be used locally to treat joint, muscle, or tendon inflammation as well as bone pain related to cancer and headache pain. Its half-life is much longer (36 to 54 hours) than that of cortisone. Also, dexamethasone is 25 to 30 times more potent than hydrocortisone (see next).

- **hydrocortisone** (Cortef®, Cortifoam®, Cortenema, Hydrocortone®)—Used to locally treat joint, muscle, or tendon inflammation as well as bone pain related to cancer and nerve compression. Injections are slowly absorbed by the surrounding tissue over a period of 24 to 48 hours. Hydrocortisone is often found as the active ingredient in various topical ointments used to reduce the inflammation of skin rashes and irritations. Its half-life is similar to that of cortisone (8 to 12 hours).

- **methylprednisolone** (depMedalone, Depoject, Depo-Medrol®, Depopred, Duralone, Medralone, Medrol®, Methapred®, Rep-Pred, Solu-Medrol®)—Used locally to treat joint, muscle or tendon inflammation, as well as inflammation from multiple sclerosis. Injections are

WHY CHRONIC STRESS IS BAD FOR YOUR IMMUNE SYSTEM

People with type A personalities (the kind of people who are "always under the gun," working 80-hour weeks, stressed all the time) have a higher risk of developing health-related problems such as heart disease. They also can develop problems with their immune systems. The body produces its own anti-inflammatory corticosteroids, namely *cortisol*. Production of this hormone by the adrenal gland is especially increased during times of psychological stress, whether it is a "normal" stress response (such as anticipating a final exam, being stuck in traffic, or being chased by a grizzly bear) or an "abnormal" stress response (such as being chronically depressed). Although the anti-inflammatory actions of cortisol can be beneficial in the short run in relieving pain and inflammation, the increases in overall cortisol production in chronically stressed individuals can actually damage the immune system. Cortisol and other corticosteroids suppress the immune system by killing off immune cells and also prevent them from passing from the circulatory and lymphatic systems to a site of infection or injury. So, while cortisol or other steroids may eliminate immune cells and relieve pain temporarily from a tender knee or wrist (especially by local injection), a "global" increase in the levels of cortisol throughout the body over a long period of time will have the negative effect of causing the immune system to "waste away." People who suffer from this problem will have their wounds heal slowly, will be more vulnerable to infections by bacteria and viruses, may have more frequent allergies, and may even have a decreased ability to fight off certain cancers.

slowly absorbed by the surrounding tissue over 24 to 48 hours. Its half-life is slightly longer than that of cortisone and hydrocortisone (18 to 36 hours).

- **prednisolone** (Delta-Cortef®, Hydeltra®, Hydeltrasol®, Key-Pred, Nor-Pred, Pediapred®, Predalone, Predate, Predcor, Predicort, Prelone®)—Used locally to treat joint, muscle, or tendon inflammation as well as cancer pain. Injections are slowly absorbed by the surrounding tissue over 24 to 48 hours. Its half-life is 18 to 36 hours.

- **prednisone** (Deltasone®, Meticorten®, Orasone®, Prednicen®, Sterapred®)—Used locally to treat joint, muscle, or tendon inflammation as well as cancer pain. Injections are slowly absorbed by the surrounding tissue over 24 to 48 hours. Its half-life is 18 to 36 hours. Prednisone is metabolized by the liver to form prednisolone (see above).

6

Herbal Remedies

A quick trip down the supplements aisle of your local health food store or pharmacy will show you that there is no shortage of herbal remedies for almost any kind of ailment—from insomnia to obesity to failing memory to persistent pain. For some people, these herbal medicines can work wonders. For others, they provide little relief— and may even be harmful. The fact is that, to date, herbal remedies for pain have not been studied and investigated scientifically, although in recent years an increasing number of scientific articles have been published on herbal products. One factor that inhibits the scientific study of herbal pain remedies is that many herbs contain dozens, sometimes hundreds, of different ingredients, so it is difficult to determine precisely which molecule in the herb is working to relieve the pain or inflammation. Another factor that limits the usefulness of herbal pain remedies is that there is no government body in the United States that regulates the amount of active ingredients in such herbs. So, whereas some herbs may contain very little of whatever active ingredient relieves pain, other herbs may contain toxic amounts of that ingredient.

Although there are too many pain-relieving herbs to cover in just one chapter, following is a brief description of the more popular herbal remedies for pain.

- **Aloe vera**. The aloe vera plant (Figure 6.1) was originally found in the wild in Africa and Madagascar, but now it is grown on almost all continents of the world. The leaves of the aloe vera plant are packed with in a clear jelly-like substance that is

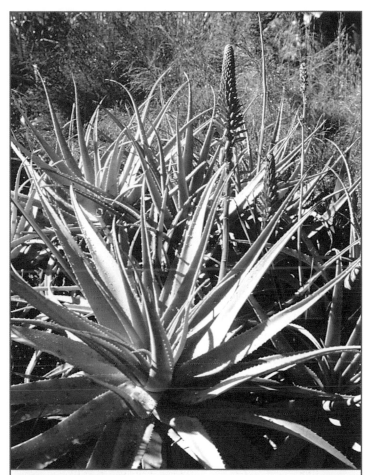

Figure 6.1 The gel in the leaves of the aloe vera plant, pictured here, is often used to relieve the discomfort of sunburns and minor cuts and scrapes.

used to make various gels, lotions, creams, sprays, and ointments. Aloe vera is widely and commonly used as a topical pain reliever for sunburns, cuts, scrapes, and other skin irritations. Aloe vera acts to reduce inflammation, swelling, and itching by inhibiting the actions of thromboxanes, bradykinins, and prostaglandins, which are molecules in the body that increase the number of pain signals sent to the brain. Aloe vera also appears to speed healing of wounds by increasing blood flow to the wound. The plant is also used to treat the painful symptoms of shingles and psoriasis. Side effects and allergic reactions to aloe vera topical preparations are quite rare. (Note: Do not confuse topical aloe vera preparations with aloe vera *latex*, which is a potent laxative!)

- **Arnica**. This plant (whose botanical name is *Arnica montana*), blooms bright yellow daisy-like flowers. It is native to Europe and Russia, but is now grown in North America and other continents. Extract of arnica is sold in the form of various creams, gels, ointments, teas, tablets and capsules. The main active ingredients in arnica are called sesquiterpene lactones, which act as counterirritants to relieve pain, inflammation, and swelling associated muscle strains and arthritis. However, when small amounts of arnica are taken internally, they can cause increases in blood pressure and heart rate, liver failure, as well as vomiting and diarrhea. Arnica should not be applied to open wounds, from which it can readily enter the bloodstream. High doses of arnica may be fatal. The risks of using arnica as a pain reliever may outweigh its potential benefits.

- **Capsaicin** (cap-say'-i-sin). Also called capsicum, capsaicin is the main ingredient found in many hot peppers (Figure 6.2) and spices such as paprika and cayenne pepper. Capsaicin is also the active ingredient in self-defense products such as pepper spray. Capsaicin directly activates nociceptors located on nerve fibers, and thus it would seem to be counterproductive (if not crazy) to apply such a substance on a wound to relieve pain. However, it turns out that capsaicin creams, gels, and lotions are indeed effective pain relievers and counterirritants when applied topically to the skin.

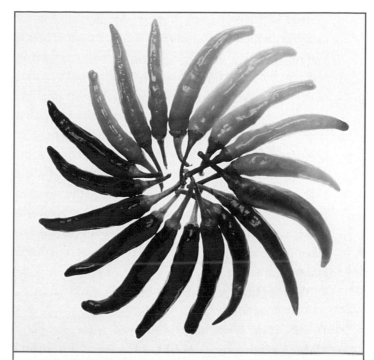

Figure 6.2 Capsaicin is the ingredient in various peppers that makes them extremely "hot" to taste, but capsaicin can also be an effective pain reliever.

The first application usually results in intense skin irritation, but subsequent applications begin to desensitize (reduce the activity of) the nociceptors located on nerve endings, eventually reducing pain signals and decreasing inflammation (caused by an interference with COX enzyme activity). Capsaicin is used to treat different types of pain, including arthritis, neuropathy (pain from nerve damage; see Chapter 4), and even postsurgical pain.

- **Chondroitin** (kon-droy'-tin). A natural component of cartilage, the tough tissue that cushions joints, chondroitin has the ability to block the enzymes that destroy cartilage tissue, thereby slowing the loss of cartilage, which is commonly seen in osteoarthritis sufferers. It also improves cartilage water retention and maintains cartilage elasticity. Chondroitin sulfate tablets, capsules, and powders are often sold in combination with *glucosamine,* another substance that improves cartilage health. Together, chondroitin and glucosamine help relieve pain and increase joint mobility in people with osteoarthritis. Since it is not a COX inhibitor, chondroitin does not cause the stomach irritation and gastrointestinal (GI) problems that aspirin and other NSAIDs cause. However, chondroitin must be taken for at least 1 to 2 months before its anti-arthritis effects can be felt. Side effects of chondroitin are rare and usually involve an upset stomach.

- **Devil's claw.** This herb is derived from the plant *Harpagophytum procumbens* ("Harpago" for short) found in the deserts of Africa (Figure 6.3). The root of this plant is cultivated, dried, chopped up, and made into capsules, powder, liquid, or tea. A limited number of studies indicate that devil's claw decreases pain and increases mobility in people who suffer from osteoarthritis—scientists are unsure exactly how. Other studies suggest devil's claw may also relieve back pain, but these findings have been inconsistent. The herb is generally well tolerated, but some side effects can include headache, ringing in the ears, stomach ulcers, loss of taste and appetite, and diarrhea. Devil's claw also acts as a blood thinner and should not be taken with other medications such as NSAIDs. The safety of long-term use of devil's claw is unknown.

- **Evening primrose oil.** This oil is extracted from the seeds of the evening primrose wildflower plant,

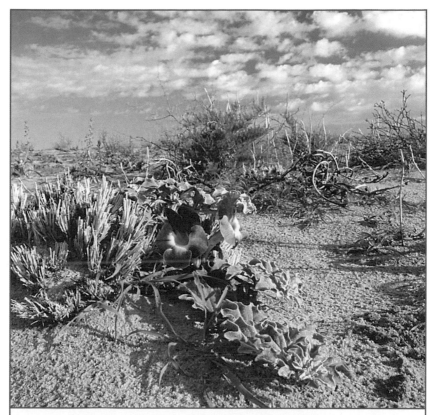

Figure 6.3 Devil's claw is found primarily in the African deserts. The dried root is said to reduce the pain of osteoarthritis, although researchers are not sure how the herb works.

Oenothera biennis, whose flowers open in the evening. The plant is native to North America, Europe, and Asia. Evening primrose oil contains essential fatty acids called linolenic acids, such as gamma-linolenic acid (GLA). GLA is involved in the formation of prostaglandins. Some scientists believe taking evening primrose oil balances the production of "good" prostaglandins (which maintain a healthy stomach lining and blood clotting) with the production of "bad" prostaglandins (which cause pain and inflammation). Evening primrose oil can be used to relieve menstrual cramps, reduce arthritis-related joint pain and swelling, and relieve pain from neuropathies (pain from damaged nerves). It can be taken in pure oil form or in oil-filled softgels or capsules. Side effects of this oil are rare and are usually experienced as an upset stomach or bloating. However, evening primrose oil may cause seizures in people with schizophrenia who are taking certain types of psychiatric medications.

- **Feverfew.** The feverfew plant (*Tanacetum parthenium*) grows wild throughout Europe and South America. The leaves of the plant are dried and chopped or ground into a powder, which can then be made into pills and capsules. Some people even chew the dried leaves, but this can irritate the mouth. Feverfew has gained recent attention for its ability to reduce the frequency and severity of migraine headaches and some of the associated symptoms, such as nausea. However, feverfew does not reduce the intensity of a migraine once it has already started. The plant has also been reported to relieve menstrual cramps. The main ingredient in feverfew was originally thought to be a substance called parthenolide, but more recently numerous active ingredients were discovered in this herb. These ingredients can inhibit the release of serotonin from blood and nerve cells and can also inhibit the synthesis of prostaglandins. Feverfew is considered a blood thinner and should not be taken with other blood thinners such as aspirin or other NSAIDs. People who are allergic to various plants, such as daisies, marigolds, or chrysanthemums, may experience an allergic reaction to this herb. Feverfew must be taken for several weeks before it becomes effective, and if a person suddenly stops taking it, he or she may suffer withdrawal symptoms and a recurrence of severe headaches.

- **Ginger**. The ginger plant (*Zingiber officinale*) is a natural spice with a pungent taste whose use in cooking and medicine can be traced back to ancient times. Early physicians found it effective in treating upset stomachs, and even today ginger, taken in the form of ginger ale, is used to ease indigestion and nausea. Ginger is primarily cultivated in tropical and semitropical areas such as Southeast Asia and Jamaica. Aside from its ability to quell an upset stomach, it is an anti-inflammatory agent that reduces the formation of prostaglandins. Ginger is mildly effective in treating various forms of arthritis. It can be taken in the form of a pill, powder, whole ginger root, tea, and—an American favorite—ginger ale. Very few people report side effects from taking ginger, and, aside from other blood thinners such as aspirin and other NSAIDs, few other drugs interact negatively with the herb.

- **Kava**. Also called kava-kava, this herb is derived from the root of the plant *Piper methysticum*, which is grown primarily in the islands of the South Pacific. Kava powder is often mixed into drinks to produce a significant sense of well-being and relaxation. Kava leaves can be chewed for a mild euphoric effect, and other forms of kava include tablets and capsules. In addition to its reported ability to reduce tension and anxiety, kava has muscle relaxant properties that relieve muscle aches. Kava may even possess local anesthetic properties similar to those of drugs like benzocaine (see Chapter 5). However, sporadic reports of kava-induced liver toxicity have caused many government agencies to keep kava on its watchlist of dangerous natural products, although no restriction against the drug has officially been legislated in the United States. Because too much acetaminophen can also cause liver damage, experts warn against taking kava with products such as Tylenol. Kava has potent effects on the brain and should not be taken in combination with alcohol, sedatives, antidepressants, or other psychiatric medications. Kava can also cause a mild upset stomach and can worsen the symptoms of Parkinson's disease.

- **Lavender**. The lavender plant (*Lavandula angustifolia*) is native to the Mediterranean region and has an intense pleasant aroma often used in soaps, perfumes, fragrances, potpourri, and air fresheners. Various lavender oils, flowers, and leaves can be applied topically to the skin for the relief of pain from sunburn and minor cuts and scrapes. Although the main active ingredient of lavender is not yet known, it can also be mildly sedating and can help treat insomnia and anxiety. However, because of this, lavender can interact with prescription sedatives, sleep aids, and opiate narcotic pain relievers. In some people, topical application of lavender can cause an allergic skin reaction.

- **St. John's wort**. The St. John's wort plant (*Hypericum perforatum*; Figure 6.4) is an increasingly popular herbal supplement that proponents claim has the ability to cure a vast array of ailments. St. John's wort appears to boost the release of the neurotransmitter serotonin in the brain, which may be the reason it is able to treat anxiety and depression. The herb contains numerous substances, two of which, hypericin and hyperforin, may be key active ingredients. St. John's wort appears to be effective in relieving the muscle pain associated with fibromyalgia and the tissue pain associated with hemorrhoids. The herb comes in tablet, capsule, cream, and ointment forms and must be taken for several weeks before it takes full effect. St. John's wort should not be taken with antidepressants such as

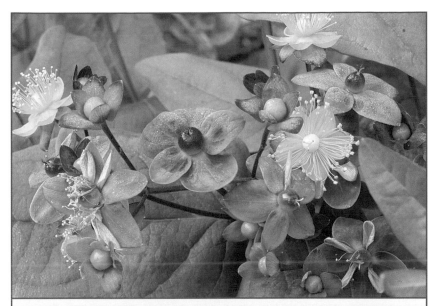

Figure 6.4 The St. John's wort plant, pictured here, is a popular herbal supplement. In some people, it relieves the symptoms of anxiety and depression, as well as muscle pain attributed to fibromyalgia.

Prozac and Zoloft. It may also reduce the effectiveness of some HIV medications. Mild side effects of St. John's wort include fatigue, dry mouth, increased sensitivity to the sun, and gastrointestinal problems.

- **Turmeric**. Turmeric (*Curcuma longa*) is a member of the ginger family and has traditionally been used as a spice that adds flavor and color to mustard and curry powder. It comes from India and southern Asia, where the stalk of the plant is scalded, dried, and made into a powder, tablet, capsule, ointment, cream, lotion, or tea. The best-characterized ingredient of turmeric is a substance called curcumin. Curcumin is an antioxidant that also causes certain cells in the body to release steroids such as cortisol, which help fight inflammation (see Chapter 5). Turmeric is used to treat arthritis, carpal tunnel syndrome, and other joint inflammations. It can cause mild side effects such as upset stomach or ulcers when used for prolonged periods of time. Turmeric is also a blood thinner and should not be taken in combination with NSAIDs such as aspirin.

- **Willow bark**. The bark of the white willow tree (*Salix alba*) has been used as a pain and fever reducer for centuries. The main active ingredient in willow bark is salicin, which the body converts to salicylic acid, a substance that acts like aspirin. In fact, the first stable form of aspirin (acetylsalicylic acid) was made from a related herb called meadowsweet. Salicylic acid inhibits

MARIJUANA—THE FORBIDDEN HERBAL PAIN RELIEVER

In recent years, a furious debate has erupted over the legality and ethical use of "medical marijuana"—that is, the use of marijuana to ease medical problems such as glaucoma, nausea associated with cancer chemotherapy, and chronic pain. It has been known for centuries that marijuana and related substances (termed *cannabinoids* [can-ah'-bih-noydz] after the botanical name of the marijuana plant, *Cannabis sativa*) are extremely effective in reducing pain. As early as 2600 B.C., the Chinese emperor Huang Ti advocated the use of marijuana for the relief of cramps and menstrual pain. In the early 1990s, scientists discovered that the body has its own cannabinoid-like pain reliever called *anandamide*. Cannabinoids, whether from marijuana or from the body's own pain-relieving system, act within the central nervous system to inhibit the transmission of pain signals.

But there is one major problem—marijuana is illegal in the United States and most other countries because of its intoxicating the formation of prostaglandins in the body, which results in reduced stimulation of nociceptors and reduced perception of pain. The salicin in willow bark may take longer than aspirin to take effect, but it may actually provide longer-lasting pain relief. In addition, willow bark does not cause the upset stomach and ulcers that aspirin can. Willow bark comes in liquid, capsule, tablet, and powder forms and is primarily taken to relieve mild-to-moderate back or muscle pain or menstrual cramps and to control the discomfort associated with arthritis. To avoid the risk of gastrointestinal side effects, ringing in the ears, and blood thinning, willow bark should not be taken with aspirin or other NSAIDs.

and potentially addictive properties. Nonetheless, in rare instances, doctors still prescribe marijuana cigarettes or capsules containing synthetic cannabinoids to people who desperately need it for the relief of pain that doesn't respond to NSAIDs, opiates, or traditional pain relievers. Medical marijuana use has created a storm of controversy among medical professionals, marijuana legalization activists and prohibitionists, and local, state, and federal governments, with patients seeking relief from chronic pain caught in the middle.

Today, scientists continue to try to unravel the biological mechanisms by which cannabinoids relieve pain, with hopes that one day a synthetic cannabinoid drug will be produced that can be legally prescribed to alleviate pain and suffering in people with AIDS, cancer, and other illnesses that cause chronic pain. At the same time, scientists hope that this new cannabinoid pain reliever will be free of the negative effects of marijuana, which include intoxication and addiction.

Appendix A

DEA Classification of Pain Relievers

In 1970, the U.S. government passed the Controlled Substances Act, which classified all drugs into one of five categories, or "schedules." In effect, this law classified drugs according to how medically useful, safe, and potentially addictive they are. These schedules are defined as follows:

SCHEDULE I   The drug or other substance has:

> ➤ A high potential for abuse.

> ➤ No currently accepted medical use in treatment in the United States.

> ➤ A lack of accepted safety for use of the drug or other substance under medical supervision.

SCHEDULE II   The drug or other substance has:

> ➤ A high potential for abuse.

> ➤ A currently accepted medical use in treatment in the United States or a currently accepted medical use with severe restrictions.

> ➤ Abuse of the drug or other substances may lead to severe psychological or physical dependence.

SCHEDULE III   The drug or other substance has:

> ➤ A potential for abuse less than the drugs or other substances in Schedules I and II.

> ➤ A currently accepted medical use in treatment in the United States.

> ➤ Abuse of the drug or other substance may lead to moderate or low physical dependence or high psychological dependence.

SCHEDULE IV	**The drug or other substance has:**
	➤ **A low potential for abuse relative to the drugs or other substances in Schedule III.**
	➤ **A currently accepted medical use in treatment in the United States.**
	➤ **Abuse of the drug or other substance may lead to limited physical dependence or psychological dependence relative to the drugs or other substances in Schedule III.**
SCHEDULE V	**The drug or other substance has:**
	➤ **A low potential for abuse relative to the drugs or other substances in Schedule IV.**
	➤ **A currently accepted medical use in treatment in the United States.**
	➤ **Abuse of the drug or other substance may lead to limited physical dependence or psychological dependence relative to the drugs or other substances in Schedule IV.**

Appendix A

Common Pain Relieving Drugs and Their Schedule Designation

Many of the pain relievers described in this book are currently classified into these schedules, as listed in the table below. However, scheduling of individual drugs can change over time as trends in abuse potential and addiction to a particular drug change. Thus, the classification of drugs is continuously updated by the Drug Enforcement Administration (DEA).

SCHEDULE	EXAMPLES OF PAIN RELIEVING DRUGS
NONE	All over-the-counter pain relievers (i.e., aspirin, acetaminophen, ibuprofen, naproxen, etc.), prescription antidepressants, anticonvulsants, muscle relaxants (except benzodiazepines), migraine medications, steroids, celecoxib, BoTox, herbal remedies, tramadol, local "caine" family (except cocaine)
SCHEDULE I	Fentanyl (depends on dose)
SCHEDULE II	Certain barbiturates, cocaine, codeine, codeine + acetaminophen (depends on dose and formulation), fentanyl (depends on dose), hydrocodone, hydromorphone, meperidine, methadone, morphine (depends on combination with other pain relievers), oxycodone, propoxyphene
SCHEDULE III	Certain barbiturates, codeine + acetaminophen (depends on dose and formulation), hydrocodone + acetaminophen, morphine (depends on combination with other pain relievers)
SCHEDULE IV	Certain barbiturates, benzodiazepines (e.g. clonazepam, Valium)
SCHEDULE V	Codeine + acetaminophen (depends on dose and formulation)

Common Over-the-Counter Pain Relievers:

SUBSTANCE	BRAND NAME
ASPIRIN:	Acuprin Bufferin Bayer Ecotrin Empirin Halfprin Healthprin St. Joseph
ACETAMINOPHEN:	Anacin-3 Bromo-Seltzer Datril FeverAll Panadol Tylenol
IBUPROFEN:	Advil Cramp End Motrin Motrin IB Midol Excedrin Nuprin
NAPROXEN:	Aleve Anaprox Naprelan Naprosyn
COMBINATION:	Excedrin (acetaminophen, aspirin, caffeine) Excedrin Migraine (acetaminophen, aspirin, caffeine) Vanquish (acetaminophen, aspirin, caffeine)

Appendix C

Acupuncture: An Alternative Method for Pain Relief

Although not a drug, acupuncture is a centuries-old method for relieving pain and other ailments that is growing increasingly popular in today's culture. The history of acupuncture has been traced back as far as the Stone Age, when stone knives and pointed rocks were used to help relieve pain. The method originated in ancient China over 4,000 years ago but wasn't introduced to the West until the 1970s when President Richard Nixon, along with a reporter for the *New York Times*, traveled to China and witnessed an appendectomy surgery that was performed using acupuncture as the sole anesthetic.[1]

The method of acupuncture was originally developed on the theory that there are channels (called "meridians," of which there are 14 to be exact) and specific points in the body through which mental, physical, and spiritual energy (which the Chinese call *Qi*, pronounced "chee") flows. When the flow of Qi through these channels and points is disrupted, the Chinese theorize that pain and illness result. In order to correct the flow of Qi, very fine sterile needles inserted into specific points of the body reestablish the flow of Qi and balance the opposing forces of nature known as yin and yang.

When acupuncture needles are inserted into the skin, the patient feels a slight sensation of touch, but no pain (if there is pain, the needle is likely in the wrong place). Once inserted, the acupuncturist can manipulate the needles by rotating or vibrating them to achieve the desired effect, or may simply leave the needles in the skin for a set period of time. Most often, when acupuncture is used for the relief of pain, small wires are connected to the needles to deliver small electrical impulses (usually only a few microamps and at a frequency of 5–2000 Hertz (impulses per second). Higher frequencies are used for major surgical procedures, whereas lower frequencies are used for general pain relief.

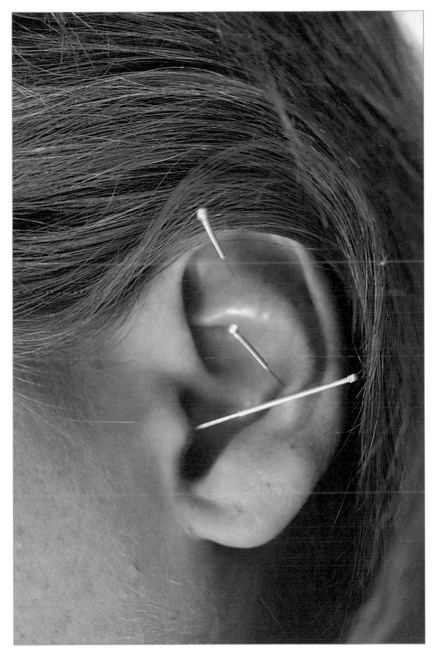

Acupuncture, an ancient Chinese form of pain relief, involves placing needles at specific points on the body.

Appendix C

Acupuncture is primarily used as a local anesthetic for back, shoulder, or neck pain; headaches; arthritis; carpal tunnel syndrome; and other ailments such as infertility, menopause, ear infections—even drug addiction. The procedure is remarkably effective, showing substantial pain relief in at least 80% of people who try it. Some hospitals, primarily those in the Far East, use acupuncture as an anesthetic for major abdominal or cardiothoracic surgeries. Some of the advantages of acupuncture are that it is safer than general anesthetics (since it does not disrupt breathing or cardiovascular functioning), allows faster post-operative recovery, and is very inexpensive. One disadvantage, however, is that acupuncture does not relax the skeletal muscles of the body and makes abdominal surgical procedures very difficult. In addition, acupuncture is not yet accepted enough in the West as a valid medical procedure (the FDA currently classifies it as an "investigational" device), and is therefore not covered by most insurance companies. Acupuncturists are usually licensed independently by specialized acupuncture schools, but some states in the United States require a medical degree in order to practice acupuncture legally.

From a biological point of view, how does acupuncture actually work to relieve pain? Currently, scientists and physicians have no idea. There is, however, no shortage of theories on the physiological basis of acupuncture. Some believe that acupuncture stimulates the release of endorphins and neurotransmitters such as serotonin and norepinephrine from nerve cells, which act to dull pain sensations (as described elsewhere in this book). Another popular theory is the "Gate Theory," which states that the insertion of needles sends many nerve signals to the spinal cord, in essence overloading it with signals causing the sensory nerves in it to shut down and thus inhibit the flow of pain signals to the brain. For other ailments, acupuncture is thought to enhance the overall functioning of the immune system and to cause blood vessel dilation, increasing blood flow to specific areas of the body.

1. Pacholyk, A. "The Biomedical Basis of Holistic Acupuncture." Available at *http://www.peacefulmind.com*.

Bibliography

Ariniello, Leah. "Migranes and Serotonin Receptors." *Society for Neuroscience: Brain Briefings*. Available online at *http://web.sfn.org/content/Publications/ BrainBriefings/migrane.html*.

———. "Cannabinoids and Pain." *Society for Neuroscience: Brain Briefings*. Available online at *http://web.sfn.org/content/Publications/BrainBriefings/ cannabinoids.html*.

Ballantyne, J., and C. A. Warfield, eds. "What to do About Pain." (Special Health Report). Digital Publication: Harvard Health Publications (April 1, 2004).

Bayer. "The History of Aspirin." Available online at *http://www.bayeraspirin .com/press/factsheets/aspirin_history.pdf*.

Chemical Heritage Foundation. "A Festival of Analgesics." Available online at *http://www.chemheritage.org/EducationalServices/pharm/asp/asp08.htm*.

Drug Information Online. "Prescription Drugs—Information, Side Effects, Interaction." Available online at *http://www.drugs.com*.

Erowid.org. "Opium Timeline." *Erowid Opiates Vault*. Available online at *http://www.erowid.org/chemicals/opiates/opiates_timeline.php3*.

Evans, P., F. Hicklebridge, and A. Clow. *Mind, Immunity and Health*. New York: Free Association Books, 2000.

Harvard Women's Health Watch. 11(June 2004): 2–3.

Julius, D., and A. I. Basbaum. "Molecular Mechanisms of Nociception." *Nature* 413 (September 2001): 203–210.

Migraine Awareness Group: A National Understanding for Migraineurs. "Migraine Awareness Group MAGNUM." Available online at *http://www.migraines.org*.

National Reye's Syndrome Foundation, Inc. Available online at *http://www.reyessyndrome.org*.

Neurologychannel. "Chronic Pain." *neurologychannel*. Available online at *http://www.neurologychannel.com/chronicpain*.

"Nonmedical Use of Prescription Pain Relievers." *Substance Abuse and Mental Health Services Administration (SAMSA), Office of Applied Studies*. May 21, 2004. Available online at *http://www.oas.samhsa.gov/2k4/pain/pain.cfm*.

"The Plant of Joy." *A Brief History of Opium.* Available online at *http://www.opiates.net.*

Professional's Handbook of Drug Therapy for Pain. Springhouse, PA: Springhouse Corporation, 2001.

Veteran's Health Administration: Office of Quality and Performance. "Local Anesthetics: Pharmacologic, Pharmacokinetic, and Clinical Characteristics." *Management of Postoperative Pain.* Available online at *http://www.oqp.med.va.gov/cpg/PAIN/pain_cpg/content/Pharmac/tableLA2.htm.*

Wall, P. *Pain: The Science of Suffering.* New York: Columbia University Press, 2000.

WholeHeathMD. "Supplements Index." *WholeHealthMD: The Source For Alternative Medicine, Complementary Medicine, Integrative Medicine.* Available online at *http://www.wholehealthmd.com/refshelf/items_index/1,1538,HS,00.html.*

Further Reading

Ballantyne, Jane, ed. *The Massachusetts General Hospital Handbook of Pain Management*, 2nd ed. Philadelphia : Lippincott Williams & Wilkins, 2002.

Rome, Jeffrey, ed. *Mayo Clinic on Chronic Pain*, 2nd ed. Rochester, MN: Mayo Clinic, 2002.

Singer, Jeffrey A. "Acupuncture—A Brief Introduction." Available online at *http://www.acupuncture.com/Acup/Acupuncture.htm.*

Warfield, C. A., and Hilary J. Fausett, eds. *Manual of Pain Management*, 2nd ed. Philadelphia: Lippincott Williams & Wilkins, 2002.

http://www.painmed.org
American Academy of Pain Medicine

http://www.theacpa.org
American Chronic Pain Association

http://www.ampainsoc.org
American Pain Society

http://www.aspirin.com
Bayer HealthCare: Aspirin

http://www.pain.com
Dannemiller Memorial Education Foundation

http://www.paincare.org
National Foundation for the Treatment of Pain

http://www.chronicpain.org
NCPOA: National Chronic Pain Outreach Association

Index

Index

Index

Picture Credits

Trademarks

Acuprin is a registered trademark of Richwood Pharmaceutical Corporation, Inc.; Adapin is a registered trademark of Fisons BV Corporation; Advil is a registered trademark of Wyeth Consumer Healthcare; Ak-taine is a registered trademark of Akorn Inc.; Alcaine is a registered trademark of Alcon Manufacturing, Ltd.; Aleve is a registered trademark of Bayer-Roche LLC; Alka Seltzer is a registered trademark of Bayer Corporation; Amerge is a registered trademark of Glaxo Group Limited Corporation; Americaine is a registered trademark of Insight Pharmaceuticals; Amytal is a registered trademark of Ranbaxy Pharmaceuticals; Anacin is a registered trademark of Insight Pharmaceuticals; Anacin-3 is a registered trademark of American Home Products; Anafranil is a registered trademark of Ciba-Geigy; Anaprox is a registered trademark of Roche Laboratories; Anbesol is a registered trademark of Wyeth Consumer Healthcare; Anestacon is a registered trademark of Alcon, Inc.; Anexsia is a registered trademark of Mallinckrodt Inc.; Arduan is a registered trademark of Richter Gedeon Vegyeszeti Gyar Rt. Corporation; Ascriptin is a registered trademark of Rorer Pharmaceutical Corporation; Asendin is a registered trademark of American Cyanamid Company; Aspergum is a registered trademark of White Laboratories; Atretol is a registered trademark of Elan Pharmaceuticals; Aventyl is a registered trademark of Eli Lilly and Company Corporation; Axert is a registered trademark of Ortho-McNeil Pharmaceutical.

Bayer is a registered trademark of Bayer Corporation; Botox is a registered trademark of Allergan, Inc.; Bromo-Seltzer is a registered trademark of Warner-Lambert Company Corp.; Bufferin is a registered trademark of Bristol-Myers Squibb Company; Butisol is a registered trademark of Wallace.

Calan is a registered trademark of G.D. Serle & Co.; Carbatrol is a registered trademark of Shire US, Inc.; Carbocaine is a registered trademark of Abbott Laboratories; Cardizem is a registered trademark of Biovail Laboratories, Inc.; Celebrex is a registered trademark of G.D. Searle & Co.; Celexa is a trademark of Forest Pharmaceuticals, Inc.; Chirocaine is a registered trademark of Chiroscience Limited LLC; Citanest is a registered trademark of AstraZeneca; Cortef is a registered trademark of Pharmacia & Upjohn; Cortifoam is a registered trademark of SRZ Properties, Inc.; Cortone is a registered trademark of Merck & Company, Inc.; CoTylenol Phenaphen is a registered trademark of McNeil-PPC; CoTylenol is a registered trademark of McNeil-PPC; Covera is a registered trademark of G. D. Searle & Co.; Cramp End is a registered trademark of Heble, Arun R.

Dalalone is a registered trademark of O'Neal, Jones & Feldman, Inc.; Damason is a registered trademark of Mason Pharmaceuticals; Dantrium is a registered trademark of Procter & Gamble Pharm; Darvocet is a registered trademark of aaiPharma; Darvon is a registered trademark of aaiPharma; Datril is a registered trademark of Bristol-Myers Company Corporation; Decadron is a registered trademark of Merck & Company, Inc.; Delta-Cortef is a registered trademark of Upjohn Company; Deltasone is a registered trademark of Upjohn Company; Demerol is a registered trademark of

Sanofi-Synthalbo Inc.; Depacon is a registered trademark of Sanofi-Synthalbo Inc.; Depakene is a registered trademark of Abbott Laboratories; Depakote is a registered trademark of Abbott Laboratories; Depo-Medrol is a registered trademark of Pharmacia & Upjohn; Dexasone is a registered trademark of Walco International, Inc.; Dexone is a registered trademark of Solvay Pharma Properties, Inc.; Dilacor is a registered trademark of Watson; Dilantin is a registered trademark of Warner-Lambert Company Corp.; Dilaudid is a registered trademark of Abbott Group of Companies; Doan's is a registered trademark of Novartis AG Corp.; Dolophine is a registered trademark of Eli Lilly and Company Corporation; Duragesic is a registered trademark of Johnson & Johnson Corp.

Ecotrin is a registered trademark of Glaxo SmithKline; Effexor is a registered trademark of Wyeth Pharmaceuticals; Elavil is a registered trademark of Zeneca Inc; E-Lor is a registered trademark of UAD Laboratories, Inc.; Empirin is a registered trademark of Burroughs Wellcome Co.; Endep is a registered trademark of Roche Products Inc.; Epitol is a registered trademark of Teva Pharmaceutical Industries; Ergomar is a registered trademark of Lotus Biochemical Corporation; Ergostat is a registered trademark of Warner-Lambert Company Corp.; Excedrin is a registered trademark of Bristol-Myers Squibb Company.

FeverAll is a registered trademark of Alpharma U.S. Pharmaceuticals Division (USPD); Flexeril is a registered trademark of Merck & Company, Inc.; Frova is a registered trademark of Vernalis Development Limited Company.

Halfprin is a registered trademark of Kramer Laboratories; Hexadrol is a registered trademark of Organon USA Inc.; Hurricaine is a registered trademark of Beutlich, L.P.; Hydeltra is a registered trademark of Merck & Company, Inc.; Hydeltrasol is a registered trademark of Merck & Company, Inc.; Hydrocortone is a registered trademark of Merck & Company, Inc.; Hydrostat is a registered trademark of Richwood Pharmaceutical Corporation, Inc.

Imitrex is a registered trademark of Glaxo Group Limited Corporation; Inderal is a registered trademark of American Home Products Corp.; Isoptin is a registered trademark of Abbott Laboratories.

Kadian is a registered trademark of US Oral Pharmaceuticals; Klonopin is a registered trademark of Hoffman-La Roche Inc.

Lamictal is a registered trademark of Burroughs Wellcome Co.; Lanacane is a registered trademark of Combe Inc.; Lidoderm is a registered trademark of Hind Health Care Corp.; Lioresal is a registered trademark of Ciba-Geigy Corp.; Lopressor is a registered trademark of Novartis Corp.; Lorcet is a registered trademark of Forest Pharmaceuticals, Inc.; Lortab is a registered trademark of UCB Phip, Inc.

Marcaine is a registered trademark of Abbott Laboratories; Maxalt is a registered trademark of Merck & Company, Inc.; Medipren is a registered trademark of River

Trademarks

West Brands, LLC; Medrol is a registered trademark of Pharmacia & Upjohn Company Corp.; Methadose is a registered trademark of Mallinckrodt Inc.; Methapred is a registered trademark of Hospira, Inc.; Meticorten is a registered trademark of Schering Corp.; Midol is a registered trademark of Bayer Corporation; Midrin is a registered trademark of Carnrick Laboratories, Inc.; Migranal is a registered trademark of Novartis AG corp.; Motrin is a registered trademark of McNeil Consumer & Specialty Pharmaceuticals; Motrin IB is a registered trademark of McNeil Consumer & Specialty Pharmaceuticals; MS Contin is a registered trademark of Purdue Frederick Co.

Naprelan is a registered trademark of Elan Corp.; Naprosyn is a registered trademark of Syntex Pharmaceuticals; Naropin is a registered trademark of AstraZeneca; Nembutal is a registered trademark of Abbott Laboratories; Neurontin is a trademark of Warner-Lambert Company Corp.; Nimotop is a registered trademark of Bayer; Norcuron is a registered trademark of Organon USA Inc.; Norpramin is a registered trademark of Merrell Pharmaceutical Inc.; Novocain is a registered trademark of Hospira, Inc.; Numorphan is a registered trademark of Endo Pharmaceuticals Inc.; Nupercainal is a registered trademark of Novartis Corp.; Nuprin is a registered trademark of Advanced Healthcare Distributors LLC; Nuromax is a registered trademark of Burroughs Wellcome Co.

Ophthaine is a registered trademark of Bristol-Myers Squibb Company; Ophthetic is a registered trademark of Allergan, Inc.; Orabase is a registered trademark of Colgate-Palmolive Company Corp.; Orajel is a registered trademark of Del Pharmaceuticals, Inc.; Oramorph is a registered trademark of aaiPharma; Orasone is a registered trademark of Solvay Pharma Properties, Inc.; Otocain is a registered trademark of Jones Pharma Incorporated Corp.; Oxycontin is a registered trademark of Purdue Pharma L.P.

Pamelor is a registered trademark of Novartis Pharmaceuticals Corp; Panadol is a registered trademark of SmithKline Beecham; Paraflex is a registered trademark of Johnson & Johnson Corp.; Parafon is a registered trademark of Johnson & Johnson Corp.; Pavulon is a registered trademark of Organon USA Inc.; Paxil is a registered trademark of SmithKline Beecham Corp.; Pediapred is a registered trademark of Fisons Corporation; Phenaphen is a registered trademark of A.H. Robins Company, Inc.; Pentothal is a registered trademark of Hospira, Inc.; Percocet is a registered trademark of Endo Pharmaceuticals Inc.; Percodan is a registered trademark of Endo Pharmaceuticals Inc.; Polocaine is a registered trademark of Astra Pharmaceutical Products, Inc.; Pontocaine is a registered trademark of Hospira, Inc.; Prednicen is a registered trademark of Central Pharmaceuticals, Inc; Prelone is a registered trademark of Muro Pharmaceutical, Inc; Propacet is a registered trademark of Lemmon Company Corp.; Prozac is a registered trademark of Eli Lilly and Company Corp.

Relpax is a registered trademark of Pfizer Inc.; Remular is a registered trademark of International Ethical Labs Corp.; Robaxin is a registered trademark of A.H. Robins Company, Inc.; Roxicodone is a registered trademark of aaiPharma.

Sansert is a trademark of Novartis AG Corp.; Seconal is a registered trademark of Ranbaxy Pharmaceuticals Inc.; Sensorcaine is a registered trademark of Astra Pharmaceutical Products, Inc.; Sinequan is a registered trademark of Pfizer Phamaceuticals, Inc.; Skelaxin is a registered trademark of Elan Pharmaceuticals, Inc.; Solarcaine is a registered trademark of Schering-Plough Healthcare Products; Solfoton is a registered trademark of Wm. P. Poythress & Co., Inc.; Solu-Medrol is a registered trademark of Pharmacia & Upjohn Company Corp.; St. Joseph is a registered trademark of McNeil-PPC; Sterapred is a registered trademark of Merz, Inc.; Sublimaze is a registered trademark of Johnson & Johnson Corp.; Surmontil is a registered trademark of Pliva, Inc.

Tegretol is a registered trademark of Geigy Chemical Corporation; Tenormin is a registered trademark of Zeneca Limited LLC; Tiazac is a registered trademark of Forest Pharmaceuticals, Inc.; Tofranil is a registered trademark of Novartis Corp.; Topamax is a registered trademark of Johnson & Johnson Corp.; Tylenol is a registered trademark of McNeil-PPC; Tylenol with Codeine is a registered trademark of Tylenol Company; Tylox is a registered trademark of Johnson & Johnson Corp.

Ultram is a registered trademark of Ortho-McNeil Pharmaceutical, Inc.; Ultram is a registered trademark of Ortho-McNeil Pharmaceutical, Inc.

Valium is a registered trademark of Roche Products Inc.; Vanquish is a registered trademark of Bayer; Vicodin is a registered trademark of Abbott Laboratories; Vicoprofen is a registered trademark of Abbott Group of Companies; VIOXX is a registered trademark of Merck & Company, Inc.

Wygesic is a registered trademark of Wyeth-Ayerst.

Xylocaine is a registered trademark of AstraZeneca.

Zanaflex is a registered trademark of Elan Pharmaceuticals; Zoloft is a registered trademark of Pfizer Inc.; Zomig is a registered trademark of AstraZeneca; Zydone is a registered trademark of Endo Pharmaceuticals Inc.

About the Author

M. Foster Olive received his Bachelor's Degree in Psychology from the University of California at San Diego, and went on to receive his Ph.D. in neuroscience from UCLA. He is currently an Assistant Professor in the Center for Drug and Alcohol Programs at the Medical University of South Carolina. His research focuses on the neurobiology of addiction, and he has published in numerous academic journals including *Psychopharmacology* and *The Journal of Neuroscience*.

About the Editor

David J. Triggle is a University Professor and a Distinguished Professor in the School of Pharmacy and Pharmaceutical Sciences at the State University of New York at Buffalo. He studied in the United Kingdom and earned his B.Sc. degree in Chemistry from the University of Southampton and a Ph.D. degree in Chemistry at the University of Hull. Following post-doctoral work at the University of Ottawa in Canada and the University of London in the United Kingdom, he assumed a position at the School of Pharmacy at Buffalo. He served as Chairman of the Department of Biochemical Pharmacology from 1971 to 1985 and as Dean of the School of Pharmacy from 1985 to 1995. From 1995 to 2001 he served as the Dean of the Graduate School, and as the University Provost from 2000 to 2001. He is the author of several books dealing with the chemical pharmacology of the autonomic nervous system and drug-receptor interactions, some 400 scientific publications, and has delivered over 1,000 lectures worldwide on his research.